MESMERISM
IN INDIA

MESMERISM IN INDIA

AND ITS

PRACTICAL APPLICATION IN SURGERY AND MEDICINE

JAMES ESDAILE

"I rather choose to edure the wounds of those darts which envy castech at novelty, than to go on safely and sleepily in the easy ways of ancient mistakings – Raleigh.

ISBN : 978-93-5324-541-2 (HB)

First Published, 1902

Published, 2020

Published by

Facsimile Publisher
12 Pragati Market
Ashok Vihar, Ph-2
Delhi-110052
E-mail: books@facsimilepublisher.com

Printed at: G. Print Process, Delhi.

Mesmerism in India

Author: James Esdaile

PREFACE TO THIS EDITION.

There is a frankness, an absence of art, about this book which makes its testimony to the power of mind over matter of double worth. No one may question the facts here recorded. They are FACTS, and they are recorded, as Truth should be, in simple speech.

It may be asked by the non-professional reader if it was necessary to present to the laity this record of the somewhat sickening surgical operations performed painlessly by Dr. Esdaile sixty odd years ago in India.

Our answer is that this is Dr. Esdaile's book, as he wrote it, and as he would wish it to be reprinted were he alive today. It will be very easy for the lay-reader to skip those portions which offend his taste. He will find sufficient other matter in these pages to repay his close attention. The Psychic Research Company has rescued this book from oblivion because it contains the simplest, clearest and most convincing data on the power of the mind to control agonizing pain.

It is nothing that we disagree with Dr. Esdaile touching the nature of the power or force manifested. To Dr. Esdaile the marvel lay in the thing—Mesmerism; in the operator, or mesmerizer. To us this book is clearest evidence of the power that lies in the subject—the mesmerized person. To the author his work was a tribute to the power of a man to help his fellow. To use it is a promise of the time to come when man shall help himself. The full importance of this collection of facts can only be appreciated when we grasp the idea that all the phenomena here produced by mesmerism are capable of reproduction by auto-suggestion. The control of pain; the restoration to health, &c., are effects which man, without the aid of another, can, and some day shall perfectly, accomplish in himself by the power of his own will while he is in a normal waking condition.

Let us honor the man who blazed the path. We have little to do now but cut away the underbrush.

SYDNEY FLOWER,
THE PSYCHIC RESEARCH COMPANY.

Chicago, May, 1902.

ENGLISH EDITOR'S PREFACE.

APPEARING before the public as the Editor of a work on Mesmerism, I trust I may be pardoned for alluding to the circumstances under which I have been called upon to undertake such a duty. Several months ago my brother, a medical officer in the service of the East India Company, surprised me by announcing that he had now found something to dispel the *ennui* of Indian life, and that his mission was to become "the Apostle of Mesmerism in India." More than twelve years ago, my attention had been arrested by reading M. Cloquet's account of his having removed a cancerous breast from a lady while in the mesmeric trance, and by his certifying her insensibility to pain. Knowing the eminence of M. Cloquet as a surgeon, and his reputation as a man of veracity, I was constrained to believe in the reality of the mysterious agent denominated Mesmerism, or Animal Magnetism; and my belief was confirmed by the fact of the operator not being a believer in Mesmerism. From that hour I never doubted that many things, scouted by most people as frauds or delusions, were merely new manifestations of this incomprehensible power. The evidence was so strong, that incredulity seemed irrational. Professional avocations hindered me paying further attention to the subject; and I had almost ceased to think of Mesmerism when it was again unexpectedly brought before me by my brother. Being thoroughly convinced of his honesty, as well as of his ability to detect imposture, I read his communications, transmitted from time to time, with the liveliest interest, and rejoiced to be at length informed that he was about to communicate his experience to the public; and that he relied on my services in seeing his work through the press, and in making any necessary alterations in the MS.

A determination to know the truth, and to afford to others the opportunity of investigating it for themselves, has induced me to read my brother's work with care, and to undertake the responsibility of preparing it for the press. In justice to him I must add, that the only alterations I have made in the MS. have been merely verbal; so that whatever merit is due to the work, either as a literary performance, or a philosophical treatise upon an imperfectly understood branch of science, none of it belongs to me.

While he will be gratified to learn that his literary offspring has assumed so little of the aspect of a changeling, by being transferred to my care, I fear that on another point he will be mortified, and that some of his readers will share in his regret. His MS. was accompanied by nine beautifully executed drawings, also intended for publication. After consulting with friends interested in Mesmerism, it has been resolved that these drawings shall not be published. They are very striking; but, unfortunately, their very fidelity is a reason for their non-publication, for, assuredly, they are fitted to shock the delicate, who are unaccustomed to witness the fearful ravages of disease on the human frame. Moreover, to publish them would add materially to the price of the work—a result which would frustrate, to some extent at least, the object of the author, who obviously desires that the British public shall have every facility in procuring information regarding the derided science of which, and with such good reason, he is so decided an advocate.

On the probable reception of the work in this country, it may be imprudent to speculate; but I cannot help hoping that the evident honesty of the writer, and his willingness to receive assistance, even from his opponents, in detecting the imposture of Mesmerism, if imposture it be, will conciliate the most incredulous, and induce them calmly to examine a multitude of facts accumulated by a man who has never been suspected to be either a knave or a fool. Every body is alike interested in fair play being afforded to the propounders of the strange facts and theories connected with Mesmerism. It is to be borne in mind, that it may be used for evil as well as for good; and that, if we obstinately refuse even to examine the subject, we expose ourselves, defenceless, to the abuse of a power capable of being perverted to the most nefarious ends. This, perhaps, will not be reckoned a fanciful danger by those who carefully peruse the author's remarks on the singular trial for the abduction of a boy. And if from this case, corroborated by the general impression in India of the frequency of far more detestable crimes, the public arrive at the conviction that Mesmerism is a terrible engine in the hands of a villain, as we have good reason for believing it to be, surely our legislators, who spend laborious nights in perfecting bills of pains and penalties against the felonious abductors of favourite poodles and the various members of the canine race, will see it to be their duty to make the practice of Mesmerism penal, save by regularly educated medical men. If my brother's book does nothing more than arouse the public to a sense of danger, it will not have been written in vain. Small as is my personal experience of Mesmerism, I have yet, with my own hands, done enough to impress me with a profound conviction that, manifold as are the blessings it confers, it must be used with care, and that it is a most formidable source of mischief in the hands of the ignorant and the unprincipled. In a note, in the body of the work, will be found an account of the influence I exerted over a young gentleman in London. I can now relate a still more striking case. When lately inviting a lady to pay me a visit, I thus wrote to her:—"Unbeliever in Mesmerism as you are, I hope to convince you of its reality by setting you asleep." In her reply she observed:—"You will, indeed, find me hard to be convinced; but if you can procure me refreshing sleep, it will be the greatest blessing, for I have not had a sound sleep for eighteen months." Knowing the anguish she had endured by family bereavements, and that her health was much impaired, a desire to relieve her sufferings made me resolve to try whether she could be brought under the influence of Mesmerism. An opportunity presented itself shortly after her arrival here. On the evening of the 9th of this month (June,) the oppressive heat of the weather rendered her languid; her voice was very rough, and she was evidently labouring under a slight attack of bronchitis. Believing that the inflammation might be subdued by means of Mesmerism, I requested permission to try its efficacy. This having been kindly granted, I subjected her to the usual manipulation for half an hour. She became perfectly placid, but did not fall asleep; she was merely drowsy, and disinclined to rise. No marked symptoms having been exhibited, I concluded that the experiment had failed; but, next morning, I was agreeably surprised to learn that she had passed a most comfortable night, and had slept for seven hours and a half without waking. Her voice also was clear, the expression of languor had left her countenance, and she felt so well that she ventured to dine at the house of a friend, distant three miles from the Manse. Whatever was the cause of the improvement, I was delighted to see my friend evidently better, and resolved again to mesmerise her. On our return from a saunter in the garden, on the evening of the 11th (June,) she lay down on the sofa, waiting the entrance of the servants to prayers. As they happened to be longer in coming than we expected, I said "Suppose I try to mesmerise you?" The reply being "Very well," I commenced my manipulations at five minutes before ten. Before that hour struck, we had the following conversation. "Oh! I am very sleepy." "Do you really think I am exerting any influence over you?" "How can I doubt it? I never felt this way before. I am in a state of the most delightful placidity."—"Why, then, I had better put off the prayers, and keep the house quiet for a little."—"No, no, don't do that. I am very drowsy," and with these words she relinquished the attempt to rise, and sank her head on the pillow. Having slipped out of the room, and ordered no noise to be made, I found her on my return still very somnolent, and, without saying another word, proceeded with my manipulations for twenty minutes. I then spoke, and, receiving no answer, proceeded to get a witness of my subsequent doings. Calling my housekeeper, I said—"Come and try if you can waken Mrs. C: I have mesmerised her, I think." She tried every means so to do, but in vain. Her respect for the lady would not allow her to obey my order to prick her with a pin; I therefore took a sharp-pointed instrument, and pricked her hand till the marks were visible. No uneasiness being manifested, I was now certain that the mesmeric sleep was established, and proceeded to test its intensity by loudly calling, and clapping my hands close to the face of the sleeper. Not a feature moved; and the exquisitely placid countenance of my entranced friend will long live in my memory.

As she was laid on a sofa in the dining-room, I could not permit her to remain there without sitting up all night to watch her, or causing my servants to do so. Circumstances rendering this inconvenient, I proceeded, at 11 o'clock, to demesmerise her. This proved a work of the greatest difficulty: for half an hour I used all the methods resorted to by the mesmerists, but with hardly any success. Being resolved, however, to break in upon her repose, I applied the strongest smelling salts to her nostrils, threw cold water on her face, and blew upon it with a pair of bellows. This rough usage roused her a little; but even after I got her to sit up, she fell helplessly into my arms, and, if let alone, would instantly have been as fast asleep as ever.

On questioning her next morning, she could give no account of what had happened. She only remembered that she lay down, and that I soon made her very drowsy. She acknowledged that I might have done with her whatever I chose, and expressed her conviction that had I amputated a limb, she would have been unconscious of the operation. What a power, then, is this for evil as well as for good! How foolish in people to expose themselves to the machinations of the wicked, by treating Mesmerism as a fraud or a delusion! *It is a fact,* proved by incontestable evidence; and capable of being applied to the relief of suffering humanity, or perverted so as to accomplish the designs of villainy. As a clergyman, I shall be happy to apply it, gratuitously for the relief of the sick, until medical men become convinced of the therapeutic value of Mesmerism, and introduce it into their practice. And for the encouragement of non-professional persons, who, like myself, are anxious to investigate the truth, I am glad to be able to state that a benevolent bishop in England, and his amiable family, are successfully employed in relieving the afflicted; and that my friend Mrs. C. expresses the warmest gratitude for the benefit she has derived from my mesmeric treatment.

The above remarks are for the general reader. I would now respectfully invite the attention of the medical profession to the facts detailed by my brother. He is neither a quack nor an enthusiast, but a regularly educated, truth-loving physician, whose reputation for talent and honesty is unquestionable. The facts he adduces cannot be controverted, and, as I was happy to learn from a medical man just arrived from Hooghly, are admitted both by Europeans and natives, on the spot where they occurred. If he, then, in eight months, has performed no less than seventy-six operations, besides relieving eighteen medical cases, how can medical men in this country justify their heartless apathy in regard to Mesmerism? It is a fact, in the highest degree disgraceful to them, that our doctors will not be persuaded even to try whether their patients can be benefitted by the mesmeric agency. They insist on going on inflicting tortures, without an attempt to ascertain whether they may not be obviated by Mesmerism. The Royal Medical and Chirurgical Society of London permitted Dr. Copland, without a word of disapprobation, to declare that "pain is a wise provision of nature; and patients ought to suffer pain while their surgeon is operating; they are all the better for it, and recover better." A London dentist has announced that several of his fraternity have resolved not to extract the teeth of persons in the mesmeric sleep! By this combination of doctors and dentists, we are threatened with the infliction of pain, whenever we are so unfortunate as to fall into their hands; and our agonies are to be soothed by Dr. Copland's pious assurance that pain is a wise infliction intended for good! Let others do as they please, for myself I shall only say, that, having twice suffered under the surgeon's knife, all the doctors in Europe shall not persuade me to permit them again to mangle my "pleasant flesh," until a persevering attempt has been made to reduce me to insensibility by means of Mesmerism. As the best persuasive to induce sufferers to form a similar resolution, I request their attention to the subjoined *resume* of my brother's mesmeric practice, as published by him in a Calcutta newspaper, on the eve of his departure for the army of the Punjaub.

It now only remains that I should publicly offer my warmest thanks to Dr. Gregory, Professor of Chemistry in the University of Edinburgh, and to Mr. Colquhoun, author of "Isis Revelata," and many other well-known works, for the highly flattering commendations they have bestowed on my brother's labours, and for many friendly and generous communications addressed to myself.

DAVID ESDAILE.

Manse of Rescobie, Forfar,
13th June, 1846.

POSTSCRIPT. 19th June.—To-day I have had a new proof of the value of Mesmerism in relieving the sick. I was visiting Isabel A——, a young woman recovering from fever; the fever had left her, but the second night before I saw her an attack of inflammation in the breast had rendered necessary the application of leeches. I found her in pain from the inflammation, and also from toothache, and complaining of inability to sleep. In ten minutes I threw her into the mesmeric trance; this was at 9 P. M.: she awoke at 2 A. M., refreshed and hungry. 23d.—The change of weather has injured my relative, Mrs. C. This evening she had a dreadful cough, which banished sleep, and gave her much pain. I proceeded to mesmerise her in the usual way: the paroxysms of the cough rendered the process more laborious than formerly; at last I succeeded in allaying the spasmodic motions of the thorax, by placing my fingers on her throat, and breathing continuously on the spot which appeared to be the seat of the irritation which annoyed her. In half an hour she was fast asleep; she slept two hours, and awoke refreshed. The cough had left her, and has not returned at this date (25th June). These are facts; and I record them for the benefit of the suffering. Let sceptics scoff, and doctors talk of danger: I have alleviated pain; and any one who will honestly make the attempt may do the same.—D. E.

TO THE

REV. JAMES ESDAILE, D. D.

My Dear Father,

However new and strange the subject of this work may be to you, I am sure that it will afford you pleasure to know that I have introduced, and I hope I may say established, a new and powerful means of alleviating human suffering among the natives of Bengal.

I shall soon ascertain to what extent other varieties of mankind are capable of benefitting by this natural curative power, as I am ordered to join the army in the field, and depart tomorrow, by dâk, a journey of eleven hundred miles!

I am, your affectionate son,

James Esdaile.

Hooghly, Feb. 1st, 1846.

PREFACE.

If this production should be unfortunate enough to attract attention *at home*, I hope that criticism will be chiefly expended upon a careful examination of the alleged *facts*, and their practical application to the improvement of Surgery and Medicine.

What I now offer to the public is the result of only eight months' mesmeric practice, in a country charity hospital; but it has been sufficient to demonstrate the singular and most beneficial influence that Mesmerism exerts over the constitution of the people of Bengal, and that *painless* surgical operations, and other medical advantages, are their natural birthright; of which I hope they will be no longer deprived.

Duty calls me to another and more extensive field, (the Civil Surgeons being ordered to join the army of the Sutlej,) where I hope to work out this curious and interesting subject in all its practical bearings, and to live to communicate my experience to the public.

Hooghly, Feb. 1st, 1846.

MESMERIC FACTS.

REPORTED BY JAMES ESDAILE, M. D.

To the Editor of the Englishman.

SIR,—Before proceeding to join the army, I have the pleasure to send you a "resume" of my mesmeric practice during the last eight months.

My experience has demonstrated the singular and beneficial influence exerted by Mesmerism over the constitution of the natives of Bengal, and that *painless* surgical operations, with other advantages, are their natural birthright, of which they will no longer be deprived, I hope.

Duty calls me to another and more extensive field, where I hope to work out this curious and interesting subject in all its practical details, and to ascertain to what extent other varieties of mankind are capable of being benefitted by this natural curative power.

I am, your obedient servant,

JAMES ESDAILE, M. D.

Hooghly, 22d Jan., 1846.

A Return showing the Number of painless Surgical Operations performed at Hooghly, during the last eight months.

Arm amputated - - - - - -	1
Breast ditto - - - - - - - -	1
Tumour extracted from the upper jaw -	1
Scirrhus testium extirpated - - -	2
Penis amputated - - - - - - -	2
Contracted knees straightened - - -	3
Ditto arms - - - - - - - -	3
Operations for cataract - - - -	3
Large tumour in the groin cut off - -	1
Operations for Hydrocele - - - - -	7
Ditto Dropsy - - - - - - -	2
Actual Cautery applied to a sore - - -	1
Muriatic acid ditto - - - - - -	2
Unhealthy sores pared down - - -	7
Abscesses opened - - - - - -	5
Sinus, six inches long, laid open - -	1
Heel flayed - - - - - - - -	1
End of thumb cut off - - - - - -	1
Teeth extracted - - - - - - -	3
Gum cut away - - - - - -	1
Prepuce cut off - - - - -	3
Piles ditto - - - - - - - -	1
Great toe nails cut out by the roots - -	5
Seton introduced from ankle to knee - -	1
Large tumour on leg removed - - -	1
Scrotal tumours, weighing from 8 lb. to 80 lb., removed 17 - - - - - -	14
Painless operations - - - -	73

A Return of Medical Cases cured by Mesmerism, during the last eight months.

Nervous Headache - - -	3	cured by one trance.
Tic-doloureux - - - - -	1	ditto.
Nervousness, and Lameness from Rheumatism of 2½ years' standing - - - - - -	1	by chronic treatment.*
Spasmodic Colic - - - - -	1	by one trance.
Acute inflammation of the eye -	1	by repeated trances in 24 hours.
Chronic ditto - - - - -	1	by chronic treatment.
Acute inflammation of testes -	1	by repeated trance in 36 hours.
Convulsions - - - -	1	by one trance.
Lameness from Rheumatism -	2	by chronic treatment.
Lumbago - - - - - -	1	by general and local mesmerising for a week.
Sciatica - - - - - -	1	ditto.
Pain in crural nerve - - - -	1	ditto.
Palsy of one arm - - - - -	1	ditto for a month.
Ditto of half the body - - -	1	ditto for 6 weeks.
Feeling of insects crawling over the body - - - - - -	1	by one trance.
	18	

It will be perceived that the above cases are chiefly diseases of the nervous system. But as sleep and the absence of pain is the best condition of the body for promoting the resolution of inflammation by the powers of Nature, I have extinguished local inflammations by keeping the patients entranced till this was effected.

*By chronic treatment is meant daily mesmerising without the intention of entrancing the patient, which is not necessary.

I beg to state, for the satisfaction of those who have not yet a practical knowledge of the subject, that I have seen no bad consequences whatever arise from persons being operated on when in the mesmeric trance. Cases have occurred in which no pain has been felt subsequent to the operation even; the wounds healing in a few days by the first intention; and in the rest, I have seen no indications of any injury being done to the constitution. On the contrary, it appears to me to have been saved, and that less constitutional disturbance has followed than under ordinary circumstances.

There has not been a death among the cases operated on. In my early operations, I availed myself of the first fit of insensibility, not knowing whether I could command it back again at pleasure.

But if the trance is not profound the first time, the surgeon may safely calculate on its being deeper the next, and when operating in public, it will be prudent to take the security of one or two preliminary trances. Flexibility of the limbs till moved, and their remaining rigid in any position we put them in, are characteristic of the trance: but there are exceptions, and these are equally diagnostic, and to be depended upon. It sometimes happens, that the limbs become rigid as they lie, and on bending them they have always a disposition to return to a state of spasmodic extension. At other times, there is a complete relaxation of the whole muscular system, and the limbs can be tossed about like those of a person just dead.

The eyes are usually closed, but the eyelids are sometimes seen a little separated, or half-open and tremulous, and the eye is even occasionally wide open, fixed, and insensible to the light. On one occasion, having ordered a man to be entranced, I returned after two hours, and was told by my assistant that the man was not affected. I went to see, and found him with half-open eyes, quivering eyelids, and trembling hands. I immediately said that he was ready, and, without further testing his condition, performed a most severe operation upon him, without his knowing anything about it.

I also wish to remark that I have seen no symptom of congestion of blood on the brain; the circulation in the trance being usually quite natural, like that of a sleeping person. My patients appear to escape the stimulating stage of the mesmeric influence altogether, and to pass at once from life to temporary death. This I am disposed to attribute to the concentrated uninterrupted manner in which the power is applied. As soon as it is felt, there is no time given to the system to rally from the first impression, and it succumbs without a struggle to the constraining power.

Some patients, when suddenly awakened. say that their vision is hazy, and their heads light; but I take this to arise from the imperfectly recovered sensibility of the brain and the organs of sense, which are not at once roused up into the full possession of their waking powers, just as is seen in persons suddenly aroused from profound natural sleep.

That the mesmeric torpor of the brain and nerves does not arise from sanguine congestion, is often beautifully seen in the first actions of persons awaking from the trance.

They open their eyes, and at the same moment recover all their faculties; but it is seen that the pupil is insensible to the light: this they also become aware of; they know that their eyes are open, and that they ought to see, but do not. The thought fills them with horror, and with a fearful cry they bury their faces in their hands, like persons struck blind by lightning; but this soon passes off, and the retina recovers its sensibility by a little rubbing of the eye. The dreadful shock given to the mind under such circumstances, or when a somnambulist awakes and finds himself standing in some strange attitude naked, in the midst of strangers (an experiment I have often made,) is a trial of the nerves which it would be very imprudent, and even dangerous, to make with any but such singularly impassive subjects as my Indian patients.

This, and the inconveniences of inducing the *mesmeric disease* (spontaneous mesmeric action in the system) by doing more than is necessary for the cure of disease, appear to me to be the real dangers to be avoided in the use of Mesmerism as a remedy.

I am now able to say from experience, that debility of the nervous system predisposes to the easy reception of the mesmeric influence, and I augur well of a patient's powers of submission, when I recognize in him the listless dejected air, "*l'air abattu,*" that usually accompanies functional debility of the nerves.

CONTENTS.

CHAPTER I.

CHAPTER II.

CHAPTER III.

CHAPTER IV.

CHAPTER V.

CHAPTER VI.

CHAPTER VII.

MESMERISM IN INDIA.

CHAPTER I.

Aversion of the old Schools and the Public to new Ideas.—Some old Notions must be suspended in fairly considering Mesmerism.—Irrational Incredulity.—Mesmerism to be tried by the usual Laws of Evidence.—Medical Men not entitled to decide the Matter for the Public.—The Public invited to judge of the Matter of Fact.—Medical Men in this Country favourably placed.—Personal Labour necessary.—All easy afterwards.—Qualifications of a Mesmeriser.—The Mesmeric Power very general.—The Sick the proper Subjects for Experiment.—The Natives of Bengal very susceptible to the Mesmeric Influence.—Nature the School of the true Physician.—Mesmerism a natural Power of Man.—Instincts of Animals.—Mesmerism known and practised in India.—Trial of Skill with an Eastern Magician.—Dangers of Mesmerism no Reason for rejecting it.—No need to interfere with the Mind in Bodily Disease.—My Patients bad Subjects for the Mental Phenomena.—The Public invited to judge the Question practically and fairly.

On the first broaching of any new branch of knowledge, there is ever a great commotion and combination among the old-established schools, which have thriven on the wisdom of their ancestors, and desire nothing more than "*stare super vias antiquas,*" satisfied with things as they are, and content to "let well alone"; and there is also a general dislike in society to have its mind unsettled, and to be called upon to think again about matters supposed to have been set at rest long ago. We have the same affection for old familiar ideas that we entertain for old coats, shoes, and hats, because they humour the peculiarities of our constitutions.

But I hope the time has at last come for the public, and the medical profession, to listen patiently to a medical man, while he relates facts that have fallen under his observation regarding Mesmerism, and for the truth of which he pledges his private and professional character, as I hereby do.

Under such circumstances, a writer has a right to expect that his statements shall be believed till they are disproved, or till dishonesty in any of the parties concerned shall be detected.

In considering a subject so new and wonderful, it will be necessary to clear away many thorns and thistles which have grown up in the mental soil, exhausting its strength, and unfitting it for receiving the seeds of truth, however freely and carefully sown. At present it will be sufficient, if, as a preliminary, the reader will dismiss the respectable old notion, that the vital powers of our bodies are confined within their own limits, and cannot be transferred to and act upon others. On the contrary, there is good reason to believe that the vital fluid of one person can be poured into the system of another, upon which it has various effects, according to constitutional peculiarities, the demand for it as a remedy, and the manner and extent to which it is exhibited in order to answer different purposes. Man is not, as commonly supposed, shut up in that pent-house, his body, isolated, and impotent to affect his fellow-creatures beneficially by a benevolent will, and his own innate resources. A merciful God has ingrafted a communicable, life-giving, curative power in the human body, in order that when two individuals are found together, deprived of the aids of art, the one in health may often be able to soothe and relieve his sick companion, by imparting to him a portion of his vitality. To believe that we possess such a power is, surely, a proud and exalting idea, which I hope the public will entertain with pleasure; and I trust to be able to prove to the satisfaction of all dispassionate and reflecting minds, that this is no fond delusion of an excited brain, but a substantial blessing, daily at work for good, extending immeasurably man's individual power of doing good by his unaided natural powers, and bringing healing and comfort to suffering humanity, all over the world.

Such is the force of habit, and aversion to a new train of thought, that this proposed extension of man's power has been received with as much distaste, as if it had been intended to deprive him of a limb, or one of his senses, and has been subjected to an irrational incredulity which nothing can satisfy. Nothing is more common than to hear persons boast, "that they will not believe it till they see it:"—some go a step farther in smothering their reason, and declare, that "they would not believe it if they saw it;"—and I have known others, not only refuse the evidence of their senses, but deny their own deeds, because they had declared the thing to be "impossible!" It is a common and ludicrous error to see people mistaking obstinacy for strength of mind, and self-sufficiency for knowledge; and aiding the delusion, by calling themselves "Sceptics," that name having once been respectable in philosophy;—whereas, they have never had any doubt about the matter, and will never condescend to hear the subject mentioned without emphatic expressions of contempt and disgust. These are the *"enfans perdus"* of knowledge, and must be left to the free indulgence of their passions and prejudices; for a man who never doubts, will never learn: he may grow older, but not wiser.

Few, in the solution of their doubts, can be privileged to the extent of St. Thomas; and the horizon of human knowledge would be miserably circumscribed, if we rejected all that we did not understand, and refused to believe facts, except on the evidence of our own senses. There is absolutely no merit in believing what we have seen and handled; this is no exercise of the judgment, and is level to the understanding of a savage: but it is the privilege of reason to be able to believe in the most surprising statements of others, if properly supported by evidence, and to adopt their conclusions, although the facts may have been observed, and the deductions drawn, by our antipodes. One such rational conversion is worth a thousand produced by crediting the senses; for its influence extends to reasoning minds all over the world. When a person says, "I would not have believed it, unless I had seen it," he must not be surprised at his neighbour requiring equal satisfaction.. As a lover of truth for its own sake, I am very little gratified by being told by my friends, "I believe it, because *you* say so." This is a very barren belief, and reaches only a small circle; our faith and opinions should be built upon a broader basis than personal confidence in any one. There are recognised laws of evidence for testing the credibility of human testimony, upon whatever subject it may be given; and however new or strange the proposition may be, we shall, by a careful and dispassionate examination of the proofs, be able to determine what we may safely believe, on what points we ought to suspend our judgments, and how much should be rejected. In spiritual matters, we have been told, "Blessed are they that have not seen, and yet have believed." This blessing also follows the ready, but discriminating, reception of truth in philosophy, morals, and secular affairs. Mental satisfaction, honour, and profit, if cared for, reward the first discoverers of the secrets of nature; riches await the men of clear sense, who know how to turn the new truths to practical purposes; and in medicine, the early application of new remedies removes much human suffering that would probably have been otherwise hopeless. It is a curious psychological phenomenon, that a hard disbelief in Mesmerism seems to be in proportion to the extraordinary facilities afforded to every one of satisfying himself by his own deeds, and the evidence of his own senses. No "*hocus pocus,*" no pretensions to exclusive powers, no attempts at concealment, are resorted to by many Mesmerisers, whose word has never been doubted, and who are well known to be neither fools nor knaves. They say to us, "Do thus, and you will probably become as wise as ourselves; or if you cannot, or will not, be at the necessary trouble,—come and see."

But people in general prefer to dictate laws to nature from their easy chairs, and amuse themselves at the expense of her followers, chasing the shapes of their own imaginations, as they are pleased to say. To those who really desire to know the truth, whatever favourite ideas it may upset, I would venture to recommend that they should examine the evidence in support of Mesmerism, just as they would any other matter worth inquiring about; and I can confidently promise that they will be richly rewarded. To encourage them, I would remind them in the words of Bacon, "that the inquiry of truth, which is the love-making or wooing of it; the knowledge of truth, which is the presence of it; and the belief of truth, which is the enjoying of it; is the sovereign good of human nature;" and that this highest gratification of humanity can only be attained by carefully training and exercising our intellect, to which the senses are only handmaids.

The public are too apt to consider the subject of Mesmerism as a professional one, and not to take the necessary means to become acquainted with it till the doctors shall have decided what is to be believed about it. This is an error on the part of the public, for, I am sorry to say, medical men in general as yet know nothing about it; and there is nothing in their previous knowledge, however great and varied, that bears upon the subject, or can entitle them to decide, *ex cathedra,* on the truth or falsehood of the new discoveries. As the question at present stands, it is one of *facts,* and of evidence in support of them, of which a jury of sensible unprofessional men can judge as well as so many doctors, to whom the subject is equally new and perplexing. When the doctors shall have experimented for themselves, or taken the trouble to witness the practice of others, and carefully studied the subject, the public cannot do better than take them for their guides; but this "consummation devoutly to be wished" is so remote, I fear, that not many of this generation will live to benefit by Mesmerism, if they wait till it is admitted into the Pharmacopœia.

I would therefore recommend the public to exercise their common sense, and sober judgment, in determining for the doctors the matter of fact; and if the community decides that it is really a remedy of great efficacy, that there is no resisting the proofs in support of it, that to know nothing about it is no recommendation to a medical man; then Mesmerism will assume its proper rank as a remedial agent, and be lodged in the hands of those who should alone practise it; for it is subject to enormous abuses in the hands of the ignorant and unprincipled. Instead of doubting and dogmatising about Mesmerism, I would earnestly entreat my medical brethren to put it to the test by personal experiment, for it is a thing to be *done*, and not talked of only: "I want *facts*, and not *words*," will be the answer of every person of common sense to the most dogmatical and ingenious objectors.

It is by medical men in this country taking up the subject experimentally, without previous knowledge of it, and having no theories to make good or defend, that the truth or falsehood of Mesmerism may be very speedily decided. By following the instructions to be hereafter given, I doubt not that many will be as successful as myself, for they are the means of putting in motion a law of nature whose springs are hidden from us, but whose effects are most wonderful and beneficial to humanity, when properly directed.

But I beg leave to warn all who have not yet a practical knowledge of the subject, that to produce the phenomena of Mesmerism is by no means a thing so light and easy as some imagine. In singularly sensitive persons the extreme degree of coma, so intense as to permit the performance of surgical operations, without awaking the patient, may sometimes be obtained in a few minutes; but, in general, it takes an hour or two, and the process often does not succeed till the second, or even fourteenth time. In this, as in everything else, nature will not "unsought be won," and only yields her secret treasures to those who court her with earnestness, sincerity, and resolution. *"Labore et sudore"* ought to be the Mesmerist's motto, until he has produced the desired results by his personal efforts, and thereby given confidence to himself and others. After this, all is easy, for any number of proper assistants may be taught to act under our superintendence;

and this is the only way in which a physician can practise Mesmerism to any extent.

But I would venture to suggest, that it will not be enough to set people to mesmerise for us by the book. It is exacting too much of human nature to expect people to sweat for hours pawing the air, &c., for our incomprehensible objects. But let them look on and see the wonderful effects produced by the labours of their superiors; and a host of willing and efficient Mesmerisers will spring up, to execute the will of the directing mind, and relieve it from the drudgery of the needful bodily exertion. Much has been written about the physical and moral qualities necessary in a Mesmeriser, and such a picture of a "perfect monster" has been drawn, that it is enough to deter one from making the attempt. If asked to select a natural Mesmeriser, I should be disposed to choose a person of a high organisation, in whom the nervous and circulating systems were equally active, with determined will, a resolution to do the thing if possible, and a love of truth and humanity, that would induce him to "do for love what gold could never buy." But, when the way has been shown, far less energy of mind and body is quite sufficient for all practical purposes. Healthy young persons, who are tractable and patient, and who will give the necessary degree of attention, can be made to work out our intentions in the most efficient manner; and I hope to make it appear that the mesmeric power is a far more general gift of nature than has hitherto been supposed. Finding it impossible, after the first month, to prosecute the subject in my own person, owing to the great bodily and mental fatigue it caused,—for I spared neither,—I set to work my hospital attendants, young Hindoos and Mahomedans; and such has been my success, that every one I have taught has become a skilful Mesmeriser. Now I do not need to mesmerise at all, having a dozen assistants to execute my wishes, whether it be in mesmeric treatment of medical cases, or for procuring coma in surgical operations.

To those who, by their own powers, may desire to test the truth for themselves, I would venture to suggest that an earnest desire to know the truth, a fixed attention, and a resolution to overcome first difficulties, are essential conditions of mind for the operator, as the means of concentrating and keeping up the continued action of the vital agent, whatever it may be. First experiments should be made on the sick, in the hope of benefitting them; which hopes, if strongly felt, will be a stimulus to exertion, and an element of success totally wanting in experimenting on healthy subjects, who are also more difficult to be affected. "The whole need not a physician, but they that are sick;" and however bountiful nature may be to her creatures, she is never prodigal, and never wastes unnecessary power. Mesmerism is the "Medicine of Nature;" and she refuses, very wisely, to take it when it is not needed; and if forced upon her in a state of health, it is very likely to do mischief; for any attempt to be better than "well" is pretty sure to make one ill. People say to me, "I would like to ascertain if I can be mesmerized; do try." I reply, "You very probably cannot; and I should as soon comply with your desire to feel the effects of opium as mesmerise you without a cause; when you need it, you will probably be benefitted by it." Besides, a person in health resisting the influence is no proof that he will remain insensible to it in an altered state of the body, when there may be an actual craving of the nervous system for this sustenance from without.

As yet, I am sorry to add, I cannot, with any degree of confidence, say who are the persons susceptible to the mesmeric influence, without first trying. But it is satisfactory to know, that by far the majority of persons acted upon by me, and my assistants, have been affected in different degrees, all of which are invaluable to their possessors, for the relief and cure of their diseases; and in most of the failures I have little doubt that we should have succeeded, if the process had been prosecuted.

The people of this part of the world seem to be peculiarly sensitive to the mesmeric power; and as it has been observed that a depressed state of the nervous system favours its reception, we can understand why they, as a body, should be more easily affected than Europeans. Taking the population of Bengal generally, they are a feeble, ill-nourished race, remarkably deficient in nervous energy; and natural debility of constitution being still further lowered by disease, will probably account for their being so readily subdued by the Mesmerist. Their mental constitution also favours us; we have none of the morbid irritability of nerves, and the mental impatience of the civilised man, to contend against; both of which resist and neutralise the efforts of nature. The success I have met with is mainly to be attributed, I believe, to my patients being the simple, unsophisticated children of nature; neither thinking, questioning, nor remonstrating, but passively submitting to my pleasure, without in the smallest degree understanding my object or intentions. How far artificial man may have forfeited his birthright I have not yet had the means of knowing; but out of the small number of Europeans who have come under my observation, the majority have also succumbed to the influence; and if the proud sons of civilisation will condescend to return for a moment to the feet of their mother Nature, they also will probably benefit by her bounties. We have so far deserted Nature, that, in return, she has renounced us as unnatural children, and left us to our self-sufficiency and artificial resources; but these, in general, are mere make-shifts and palliatives, compared with the steady and enduring curative powers of nature, when properly understood and brought into action. The whole art of the true physician is exerted to induce nature to interfere and take up the case of his patient; and when he sees signs of her gracious presence, he only reverentially looks on, and confines himself to removing impediments in her way. But the routine practitioner will rarely condescend to divide with nature the merit of the cure. He and his pills, powders, and potions, must have all the credit; and if any one pretends to be able sometimes to cure disease by the unassisted powers of nature, he is called quack, impostor, or fool, and hunted down as a *fera naturae*. But, in my estimation, the genuine medical quack is he who, professing to cure disease, yet allows his patients to suffer and perish, by ignorantly, or presumptuously, despising any promising or possible means of relief. The Father of Medicine thought very differently from his degenerate sons, for he says,—"Nothing should be omitted in an art which interests the whole world, which may be beneficial to suffering humanity, and which does not risk human life and comfort." But a time was, when apothecaries, chemists, and diploma'd physicians did not exist; when man was an unreasoning animal, devoid of all the resources of art, yet subject to all the ills that natural flesh is heir to; and it is a subject of deep interest to the philosopher and the physician to ascertain what were his natural remedies, in common with the other animals; whether his instincts were as strong as theirs, and to what conservative powers he resorted when labouring under disease. That he possessed such appears to me to be extremely probable, from the analogies of the animal creation, and the universal benevolence of the Deity to his creatures. It must be most important and instructive to discover what *were*, or, if not yet known, what *are*, the natural remedies of man; for by observing their effects we shall best understand the restorative processes of Nature, and be able to imitate them by art, with a certainty hitherto unattained by medicine.

So far from Mesmerism being a new and unnatural art, there is every reason to believe that it is the oldest and most natural mode of curing many of the severe, uncomplicated diseases of the human race. Let us imagine, for a moment, the condition of savage men, before, by long experience, they had learned to avail themselves of the medicinal virtues of the vegetable and mineral kingdoms, for the cure of their most pressing diseases. Man, in this state, would be more helpless than the brute creation; they have happy instincts, many of them known to us, by which they are directed not only to their natural food, but to their natural medicines. But man, so far as we yet know him, could in his sufferings only make vague experiments on the natural objects around him, in the desperate hope of stumbling upon some suitable remedy. This might occasionally happen, but he was more likely to be poisoned than cured by his first experiments. The very fish were more favoured than he. The salmon, by an infallible instinct, quit the sea at a certain season, and ascend the rivers, thereby getting rid of their tormentors, the sea-lice (which the fresh water speedily kills,) and at the same time reaching the spots destined for the propagation of their kind. After depositing the spawn, the parent fish, black, lank, and sick, distasteful to themselves, and unwholesome to us, hasten to the sea to renovate their health; whence, again, they issue in another year, increased in size, and brilliant as silver, to run the same course as long as life continues. The young fry, also, the moment they break the egg, turn their heads seaward, and never stop till they reach the ocean, whose action is necessary for their growth and health.

The dog eats grass, and licks his sores when sick; the cow, and calf even, sham dead, to induce the crows to pick the vermin from their eyes and ears; the chick, as soon as it breaks the shell, pecks gravel, to aid digestion; the mongoose, after being bitten by its enemy, the snake, retires to the fields, to seek its antidote against the poison; and this it finds, for it comes back quite well; and at certain seasons the wild animals resort, from the most distant parts of the country, to the "salt-licks," to renovate their constitutions. Numberless instances of the same kind will occur to the naturalist, and the humble observer of nature even; and is it imaginable that the ever-watchful, all-bountiful Providence of God should have left the "noble savage," alone of all His creatures, to run such cruel risks, and perish helplessly in his natural ignorance? Reasoning *a priori,* we should say not; and our positive knowledge of the equal care bestowed by God on all his creatures, forbids the supposition. Man, then, had probably some instinct by which he was directed to a natural medicine of sovereign virtue, and by which the hunter and his family were saved from starvation, when disease, for a time, deprived his right hand of its cunning, unnerved his iron sinews, and bowed his gallant head. If this be a natural supposition, what could be his resource if not Mesmerism—that inherent power, implanted, as I conceive, in the human being, for the solace of his suffering fellow creature? This is the simplest and most speedy restorative of the powers of life, in cases adapted to it (for, like every natural agent, it has its conditions and limits;) and men in pain have an instinctive tendency to perform the required processes. From its simplicity, how consonant with all we know of the laws of nature would be such a power, and how admirably adapted to meet the exigencies of savage life!

The more observing among savage men, it is presumable, would soon detect the latent curative powers of their bodily system, and develope them into an art for the cure of disease, and the advancement of their own interests. But when experience had given them skill, and it became a source of gain, they made, we may suppose, a mystery of their calling, and attempted to secure the lucrative secret for themselves and families. Hence, among the savage races of mankind, we see the healing art practised exclusively by conjurors, either artfully concealing the secret of their power by incantations, and other mummery, or, possibly, themselves deceived into a belief of the efficacy of such accomplishments. If the Mumbo Jumbo men of Africa, the medicine men of America, and the charmers of this country, ever succeed in relieving their patients (and here they do,) I am disposed to think that it is generally in cases curable by Mesmerism. The following extract from my "Mesmeric Journal" will show that this is not so fanciful a speculation as it may at first appear, and that Mesmerism is actually practised in this country, and has probably been so from time immemorial, like every other custom in this immutable society.

June 9th, 1845.—I had to-day the honour of being introduced to one of the most famous magicians in Bengal, who enjoys a high reputation for his successful treatment of hysteria, and had been sent for to prescribe for my patient (whose case will be afterwards given,) but came too late; the success of my charm, Mesmerism, having left him nothing to do. Baboo Essanchunder Ghosaul, deputy magistrate of Hooghly, at my request introduced me to him as a brother magician, who had studied the art of magic in different parts of the world, but particularly in Egypt, where I had learned the secrets of the great Sooleymann, from the moollahs and fuqueers, and that I had a great desire to ascertain whether our charms were the same, as the hakeems of Europe held the wise men of the East in high estimation, knowing that all knowledge had come from that quarter. I proposed that we should show each other our respective charms, and, after much persuasion, he agreed to show me his process for assuaging pain. He sent for a brass pot, containing water, and a twig with two or three leaves upon it, and commenced muttering his charms, at arm's length from the patient. In a short time he dipped his fore-finger into the water, and, with the help of his thumb, flirted it into the patient's face; he then took the leaves, and commenced stroking the person from the crown of the head to the toes, with a slow drawing motion. The knuckles almost touched the body, and he said that he would continue the process for an hour, or longer, if necessary; and it convinced me that, if these charmers ever do good by such means, it is by the Mesmeric influence, probably unknown to themselves. I said that I was convinced of the great efficacy of his charm, and would now show him mine; but that he would understand it better if performed on his own person. After some difficulty, we got him to lie down, and, to give due solemnity to my proceedings, I chanted, as an invocation, the chorus of the "King of the Cannibal Islands!" I desired him to shut his eyes, and he clenched his eyelids firmly, that I might find no entrance to the brain by that inlet. In a quarter of an hour he jumped up, and said he felt something disagreeable coming over him, and wished to make his escape. He was over-persuaded to lie down again, however, and I soon saw the muscles around the eye begin to relax, and his face became perfectly smooth and calm. I was sure that I had caught my brother magician napping, for, in a few minutes, he bolted up suddenly, clapped his hands to his head, cried he felt drunk, and nothing could induce him to lie down again; *"abiit, excessit, evasit, erupit!"* Next day I saw him, and said, "Well, you were too strong for my charm last night; I could not put you to sleep." "Oh! yes, Sahib," he answered, "you did; I allow it; it is allowed that you put me to sleep."

A gentleman, whose case will be given hereafter, immediately recognised the identity of the two processes, and told me that he had been Mesmerised, he now knew, in a different part of the country, and with much relief, in a painful affection of the leg. In addition to the traction with the leaves, his mesmeriser had breathed carefully upon the pained part, just as my assistant had done when mesmerising him locally for rheumatism. It thus appears that the beneficial effects of the Mesmeric processes are known in this country, and the secret has probably descended from remote antiquity, in certain families, or castes.—Farther on, when speaking of Somnambulism, a curious history will be given, which leads me to suspect that they knew the evil, as well as good, of Mesmerism, and practise it for the most villainous purposes. The possible evil resulting to society from the practice of Mesmerism has been a favourite objection, even when the evidence of its existence and power could no longer be resisted.

But the tendency of all power depends upon the direction given to it for good, or evil; and to eject opium, mercury, and prussic acid from the pharmacopœia, because, when injudiciously administered, they poison, instead of curing our patients; or to reject the agency of steam for the purposes of life, because it sometimes takes us a longer journey than we intended, would be as reasonable as to refuse to be cured by Mesmerism, because it could also injure us, if ignorantly and injudiciously applied. That this agent may, and will, be turned to the most diabolical purposes, is most certain, if the public will not be at the trouble to think upon the subject, and defend itself by common-sense precautions. But the power as it comes from the Creator is pure, and the perversion of it is the work of the creature. The object of man's life here clearly is—to separate the good from the evil; "to prove all things, and hold fast that which is good;" and this can be done in Mesmerism, as in anything else: the abuse, and not the use of any great power, is to be dreaded and guarded against. I have great hopes that my experiments will go far to separate the regions of mind and body, which, it seems to me, have been unnecessarily and perplexingly intermingled by former Mesmeric observers; and this will not only simplify the Mesmeric treatment of disease, but remove the principal objection to it; namely—the necessity of acting on the mind, often injuriously, during the cure of a bodily infirmity. It will appear, that in the exercise of the art, as a medical agent of the most benign as well as powerful nature, the mind has never been attempted to be influenced by me, nor has it ever been heard of in my practice. In subjecting my patients to the sanative influence of Mesmerism for bodily complaints, no mental *rapport* has ever been thought of; and if so much can be done without it, I am sanguine that it will soon be proved to be a tedious and unnecessary complication of the art, and "more honoured in the breach than the observance." In the management of mental disease, it will probably be required, and be useful, as the mind depends much more upon organisation than is generally supposed. But this is only an extension of the blessing, if the power is wielded in all honour and simplicity of purpose. In this, as in other matters, the danger lies in the company we keep. The possessor of a well-filled purse does not seek the companionship of pickpockets; and the honest man eschews the society of knaves; and if Mesmerism is thought likely to benefit us, the same commonsense mode of proceeding should influence us in the disposal of our bodies and minds, when affected by disease. I am convinced that in the majority of bodily evils removable by this means, there will be no need to interfere with the mind at all. To do so is a mere travelling out of the record; and where a mixed treatment is required it can be safely adopted, by using the simple precaution of seeking an honest man with the necessary knowledge of the subject; and let us hope that such will soon abound. Many will be disappointed that I have no mental wonders to relate; but no inference against the existence of such wonders can be fairly drawn from the silence of my patients. My researches have been purely physical, and preclude me from getting at the mind at all, for all activity of mind is the natural enemy of the purely physical impressions made upon the system; I therefore seclude the brain from all external impressions as rapidly as possible; the object being to extinguish bodily and mental sensibility together, and altogether; and in proportion to our success in effecting this, is the early inducement of Coma for surgical purposes. It is quite unreasonable to expect to extract music from a fiddle without strings: and I endeavor to break at a blow, as it were, all the strings of the mind—the five senses. It is true, that this treatment is only required for acute diseases, or to induce insensibility to pain, and it might be expected that in the treatment of chronic diseases, I should be able to elicit the mental phenomena, if they exist in nature. But as my principal object is to ascertain how far this new agent is capable of alleviating bodily suffering, I have purposely kept myself from embarking on the troubled sea of metaphysics, till the more pressing bodily problem shall be solved, and a "terra firma" of indisputable facts created, from whence we may securely, and at leisure, examine, and attempt to understand, the high and mysterious objects above us.

My patients, being the poorest and most ignorant of the people, and convicted felons from the same degraded orders, are the most unfavourable subjects for psychological experiments. As to *physique,* men are nearly the same all the world over: an universal vital law reduces all to the same level of animal, and the coolie, therefore, may be able to mesmerise the philosopher; but the difference in *morale* is so great, not only among races, but individuals, as to preclude all sympathy, and to often amount to actual antipathy, and mutual repulsion. Although in producing the physical effects of Mesmerism, I have not seen any necessity for the sympathy and *rapport* we read so much about, I can readily understand, that in eliciting the higher mental phenomena, these fine mental sympathies may be developed, and be necessary for the success of the abnormal mental manifestations; but my patients and I have probably too little in common to admit of mental sympathy between us. It will be seen, however, in the chapter on Somnambulism, that I have created a singular *bouleversement* in the minds of coolies and pariahs even, when under the Mesmeric influence.

The public, when examing a subject so deeply interesting to them, will, I hope, take an enlarged and liberal view of the matter, and look for fundamental and incontrovertible truths, which are practically important, and not allow themselves to be cheated out of their senses and judgment, by the doubtful, mysterious, and theoretical parts of the subject being exclusively dwelt upon, by those who *wish* Mesmerism to be untrue, or by others who have neither the desire nor capacity to acquire new knowledge. Errors of observation and of judgment must often occur in investigating a new and difficult subject, but I hope such unintentional mistakes will be excused; and wherever they shall be pointed out in my observations, I shall be ready to acknowledge and correct them. Let all doubtful evidence be totally rejected, and a mass of substantial important truth will remain, which, I am confident, the public "will not willingly let die;" for human nature can ill afford to lose any new and promising source of comfort to suffering humanity.

Before concluding these prefatory remarks, I beg the reader

not to do me the injustice to think me a Mesmeric doctor, for it would be as true to call me a rhubarb, jalap, or castor-oil physician. Mesmerism often comes to the aid of my patients, when all the resources of medicine are exhausted, and all the drugs of Arabia useless; and therefore, I consider it to be my duty to benefit them by it, and to assist in making it known for the advantage of mankind.

CHAPTER II.

The French Commission of 1779.—Both Right and Wrong.—The Mesmerists properly punished.—Condition required in the Patient.—State of my Mind before experimenting for myself.—Report of the Bishop of Lausanne to the Pope.—His Reply.—Accidental Nature of my First Experiment.—Accidental Nature of my Second Experiment.—First Mesmeric Surgical Operation.—Conclusion.

THE most formidable, because the most reasonable argument against the existence of Mesmerism as a natural power, is, perhaps, the report of the French Commission in 1779, of which Franklin was president. The verdict of the *Savans* was fair enough, considering the nature of the evidence placed before them; but yet, (such is human fallibility,) in this case *summum jus* was also *summa injuria;* truth was sacrificed to falsehood, as I think will clearly appear from a short analysis of their proceedings. This will probably not be time wasted, as I have heard intelligent gentlemen say, that the report of the French philosophers still decided their opinions. They had a series of axioms in Mesmerism presented to them, whose truth they were to examine, and the efficacy of certain processes was to be proved to their satisfaction by experiment.

The Mesmerist's object seems to have been, to try to convince the commission that he had a secret worth knowing, and yet continue to keep it to himself, by hiding its extreme simplicity under a load of complicated machinery and various kinds of mummery. D'Eslon, the pupil of Mesmer, propounded his laws of animal magnetism, after this fashion:—

"I. Animal magnetism is an universal fluid, constituting an absolute plenum in nature, and the medium of all mutual influence between the celestial bodies, and betwixt the earth and animal bodies."

This is only a gigantic assertion.

"II. It is the most subtle fluid in nature, capable of flux, and of reflux, and of receiving, propagating, and continuing all kinds of motion."

The first two clauses are probable enough; the last is only rash dogmatism.

"III. The animal body is subjected to the influences of this fluid by means of the nerves, which are immediately affected by it."

We see no other way, at present.

"IV. The human body has poles, and other properties, analogous to the magnet."

The first proposition has never been proved, and takes everything for granted; there is only likelihood in the second.

"V. The action and virtue of animal magnetism may be communicated from one body to another, whether animate or inanimate."

True, as regards the relations between animate bodies; and these can also impregnate inanimate substances.

"VI. It operates at a great distance, without the intervention of any body."

True.

"VII. It is increased and reflected by mirrors, communicated, propagated, and increased by sound, and may be accumulated, concentrated, and transported."

Soothing sounds may possibly assist in lulling the brain, but quiet is far more essential; the other assertions are borne out by modern experience.

"VIII. Notwithstanding the universality of this fluid, all animal bodies are not affected by it; on the other hand, there are some, though but few in number, the presence of which destroys all the effects of animal magnetism."

The first part correct, the last not improbable.

"IX. By means of this fluid, nervous diseases are cured immediately, and others mediately; and its virtues, in fact, extend to the universal cure and preservation of mankind."

True; to so great a degree, that we do not yet know how far it may go.

Is it surprising that the Commission dismissed contemptuously such a mass of sheer assertion and unsupported theory, seasoned with truth to be sure, but so diluted and obscured as not to be recognisable? Like a Bengal witness, D'Eslon was not content to tell the truth simply, but added so many corroborating inventions of his own, that no one knew what to believe, and the case was dismissed as unworthy of further investigation. He ruined himself, and his cause, also, (perhaps in ignorance, however,) by loading the truth with a parcel of trumpery machinery, through which he hoped the power of nature would nevertheless penetrate. But Nature, like an over-loaded camel, turned upon her driver, and threw him and his paraphernalia of magnetic platforms, conducting-rods and ropes, pianos, magnetised trees and buckets, into the dirt; and truth retired in disgust to the bottom of her well, there to dwell till more honest men should draw her forth again to surprise and benefit the world.

As far as my observation goes, all that is necessary for success, if the parties are in the relation of agent and subject, is *passive obedience* in the patient, and a sustained attention and patience on the part of the operator. The process being a natural one, the more the parties are *in a state of nature* the better: the bodies of my patients being naked, and their heads generally shaved, is probably of no small consequence in the proceedings.

Before presenting to the reader my first experiment in mesmerising, I may perhaps be excused the egotism of giving a brief sketch of the history of my belief in Mesmerism, as it is a remarkable epoch in a man's life the day he discovers that he possesses the temporary power of life and death over his fellow-creatures.

Ever since Dr. Elliotson declared, years ago, that he "should despise himself if he did not declare his conviction of the truth of Mesmerism," I ceased to regard it lightly, and paid attention to all well-attested reports upon the subject. At last the facts became so numerous, and were so well supported by credible witnesses, and kept their ground so firmly, both against adverse reasoning and ridicule, that I felt compelled to surrender my belief in the existence of the Unknown Power, or cease my reason and judgment. Ten days before making my first experiment, I thus wrote to a friend in England:—"What think you of this new mystery, Mesmerism? For my part, I am thinking seriously about it, and cannot help suspecting that we have hit upon one of Nature's great secrets. I keep myself perfectly neutral, and hear the *pro* and *con*. If it turns out to be a delusion, I shall be happy to assist in digging its grave."

The uniformity of the phenomena described by different persons, and coming from various parts of the world, strongly arrested my attention, and impressed me with the conviction that some new general law of Nature had been discovered. England, France, Germany, and America, all combined to give the same evidence in support of the new doctrines, or, rather, new phenomena of Nature. About the time that Miss Martineau's disclosures appeared, I also read a curious and striking document written in May, 1841, by the Archbishop of Lausanne and Geneva, and addressed to the Sacred Penitentiary, at Rome. As it may possibly make the impression upon others that it did on me, it is here transcribed.

"Most Eminent Lord,

Since that which has hitherto been answered respecting animal magnetism seems by no means to suffice, and it is much to be wished that cases not unfrequently occurring may be solved more and more uniformly, the undersigned humbly lays before your Eminence that which follows:—

"A magnetised person, who is generally of the female sex, enters into that state of sleep called *Magnetic Somnambulism* so deeply, that not even the greatest noise at her ears, nor any violence of iron or fire, is capable of raising her from it. She is brought into this kind of ecstacy by the magnetiser alone, to whom she has given consent (for consent is necessary,) either by various touches or gesticulations, when he is present, or by a simple command, and that, too, an internal one, when he is at a distance of even several leagues.

"Then, being interrogated, aloud or mentally, concerning her own disease, or those of absent persons entirely unknown to her, this person, who is evidently one unlearned, at once exhibits great superiority in science to medical men; announces most accurately anatomical matters; indicates the cause, seat, and nature of internal diseases in the human body, which, to the skilful, are most difficult of understanding, and unravels their progress, variation, and complications; and this in the terms proper to them, and prescribes the most simple and efficacious remedies.

"If the person concerning whom the magnetised woman is consulted is present, the magnetiser establishes the relation between them by means of contact. If, however, he be absent, a lock of his hair supplies his place, and suffices; for, when this lock of hair is brought into the proximity of the hand of the magnetised person, he declares what it is (without casting his eyes on it,) whose hair it is, where the person is actually sojourning, to whom the hair belongs, what he is doing, and affords the above-mentioned information respecting his disease not otherwise than if, after the manner of medical men, he were inspecting the interior of his body.

"Lastly, the magnetised person does not see with the eye. The eyes being covered, though not knowing how to read, he will read off whatever is placed on his head or stomach, whether a book or manuscript, open or shut. His words, too, seem to issue from this region: but when brought out of this state, either at the order, even internal, of the magnetiser, or, as it were, spontaneously at the moment previously announced by himself, he appears to be not at all conscious of the things gone through by him in the paroxysm, how long soever it may have lasted; what may have been demanded of him; what he may have answered; what he may have undergone; all these things have left no idea in his understanding, nor the least vestige in his memory.

"Therefore, the undersigned petitioner, seeing valid reasons for doubting whether such effects, the occasional cause of which is shown to be so little proportioned to them, be simply natural, earnestly and most fervently prays that your Eminence in your wisdom, for the greater glory of the Omnipotent, as well as the greater good of souls, which have been redeemed by the Lord at so great a price, may be pleased to decide, whether, admitting the truth of the premises, a confessor or curate may safely permit to his penitents or parishioners:—

"1. That they practise animal magnetism, endowed with such, or other like characteristics, as an art auxiliary and supplementary to medicine.

"2. That they consent to be thrown into such a state of magnetic somnambulism.

"3. That they consult persons magnetised in such a manner either concerning themselves or concerning others.

"4. Or that they undertake one of these last mentioned three things, having first taken the precaution of formally renouncing in their minds every diabolic compact, explicit or implicit, as well as all satanic interventions, since, notwithstanding such precautions, similar effects, or some such effects, have been obtained by some persons.

"Most Eminent Lord, by command of the most Rev. the Archbishop of Lausanne and Geneva, your Eminence's most humble and most obedient servant,

"James Xavier Fontana,

"Chancellor of the Episcopal Chancery.

"Friburgh, in Switzerland, Episcopal Palace, the 19th of May, 1841."

RESPONSE.

"The Sacred Penitentiary, the premises having been maturely weighed, considers that these should be answered as it now answers:—the use of magnetism, as set forth in the case, is not permissible.

"Given at Rome, in the Sacred Penitentiary, the 1st day of July, 1841. "C. CARD, Castracane, M. P.
"PH. POMELLA, of the S. P. Sec'y.

"Certified as a copy conformable to the original.—Friburgh, the 26th July, 1841.

"By order, J. Perroulaz, Sec'y. of the Bishopric."

It will be observed, that though the subject is held in dread by the reporter, as probably of diabolic origin, yet it is treated as a "great fact," known to, and believed in, by a large community, so that catholics and protestants are found alike professing a belief in Mesmerism. If the twentieth part of what was reported was true, it well deserved careful investigation; and, as I had no dread of knowing anything that God has permitted to be known, I determined to try to find out the truth for myself, on the first favourable opportunity. In choosing a proper subject to experiment upon, I should probably have selected some highly sensitive female of a nervous temperament, and excitable imagination, who desired to submit to the supposed influence. But, I beg it to be particularly remarked, my first essay was not guided by theory, and was not made on a subject supposed to be favourable. On the contrary, the very worst specimen of humanity, theoretically considered, was the person destined to be my first mesmeric victim; he being none other than a Hindoo felon of the hangman cast, condemned to labour on the roads, in irons. Accident alone determined my choice, and decided the matter for me, perhaps much better than theory would have done; for I should as soon have thought of commencing operations on the first dog or pig I met on the road, as of selecting this man for his good mesmeric "material."

There are some interesting particulars in this first successful mesmeric experiment in India, to which I beg leave to direct the reader's attention.

I. The purely accidental and unpremeditated nature of the experiment.

II. All want of consent between the parties.

III. The operator's want of belief in his own power; for I had never seen Mesmerism, and all I knew about it was from scraps in the newspapers.

IV. The absolute ignorance of the patient; it being impossible that he should ever have heard of Mesmerism.

V. The impossibility, therefore, of imitating the mesmeric phenomena.

Under all the circumstances of the case, collusion between the parties will not, I presume, be suspected: and every possible care was taken to exclude any source of fallacy in the experiment. European gentlemen, sceptical and critical, or so strong in disbelief that they would have reasoned themselves out of their senses, if they could: Ignorant Hindoos and Mussulmanns, who merely used their eyes and ears without an attempt at reflection, will all be found, by their separate and independent reports, bearing testimony to the same series of phenomena. As I might never succeed again, I endeavoured to make this case as perfect as possible in all its parts, by bringing the senses of different people to bear upon it, in all its stages; and, I must say, that I cannot see any possible opening for mistake or deception. It has for many months been before the Indian public, who were invited to point out any source of error that may have escaped me, and no attempt has been made to disprove the facts, or explain them away, except by the easy and sweeping charge of imposition in the patient, and delusion in the observers; of the probability of which I shall now give the reader the means of judging.

First Experiment.

Madhab Kaura, a hog-dealer, condemned to seven years' imprisonment, with labour on the roads, in irons, for wounding a man so as to endanger his life, has got a double Hydrocele. He was ordered to be taken from the jail to the charity hospital, to be operated upon.

April 4th.—The water was drawn off one side of the scrotum, and two drachms of the usual cor. sub. injection were thrown in. On feeling the pain from the injection, he threw his head over the back of the chair, and pressed his hands along the course of the spermatic cords, closing his eyelids firmly, and making the grimaces of a man in pain. Seeing him suffering in this way, I turned to the native sub-assistant surgeon, an *eleve* of the medical college, and asked him if he had ever seen Mesmerism? He said that he had seen it tried at the medical college, but without effect. Upon which I remarked, "I have a great mind to try it on this man, but as I never saw it practised, and know it only from reading, I shall probably not succeed."—The man continuing in the position described, I placed his knees between mine, and began to pass my hands slowly over his face, at the distance of an inch, and carried them down to the pit of his stomach. This was continued for half an hour before he was spoken to, and when questioned at the end of this time his answers were quite sensible and coherent.

He was ordered to remain quiet, and the passes were continued for a quarter of an hour longer—still no sensible effect. Being now tired (thermometer 85°,) I gave it up in despair, and declared it to be a failure. While I rested myself, the man remained quiet, and made fewer grimaces, and when ordered to open his eyes, he said there was smoke in the room. This roused my attention, and tempted me to persevere. I now breathed on his head, and carried my hands from the back of his head over his face and down to the epigastrium, where I pressed them united. The first time this was done, he took his hands off his groins and pressed them both firmly down upon mine; drew a long breath, and said, "I was his father and mother, and had given him life again." The same process was persevered in, and in about an hour he began to gape, said he must sleep, that his senses were gone; and his replies became incoherent. He opened his eyes, when ordered, but said he only saw smoke, and could distinguish no one; his eyes were quite lustreless, and the lids were opened heavily. All appearance of pain now disappeared; his hands were crossed on his breast, instead of being pressed on the groins, and his countenance showed the most perfect repose. He now took no notice of our questions, and I called loudly on him by name without attracting any notice.

I now pinched him, without disturbing him, and then asking for a pin in English, I desired my assistant to watch him narrowly, and drove it into the small of his back; it produced no effect whatever; and my assistant repeated it at intervals in different places as uselessly. His back had continued to arch more backwards latterly, and he now was in a state of "opisthotonos;" the nape of his neck resting on the sharp back of the chair, and his breech on the edge of it. Being now satisfied that we had got something extraordinary, I went over to the Kutcherry, and begged Mr. Russell, the judge, and Mr. Money, the collector, to come and see what had been done, as I wanted the presence of intelligent witnesses in what remained to do. We found him in the position I had left him in, and no hallooing in his ears could attract his attention. Fire was then applied to his knee, without his shrinking in the least; and liquor ammoniæ, that brought tears into our eyes in a moment, was inhaled for some minutes without causing an eyelid to quiver. This seemed to have revived him a little, as he moved his head shortly afterwards, and I asked him if he wanted to drink; he only gaped in reply, and I took the opportunity to give, slowly, a mixture of ammonia so strong that I could not bear to taste it; this he drank like milk, and gaped for more. As the "experimentum crucis," I lifted his head, and placed his face, which was directed to the ceiling all this time, in front of a full light; opened his eyes, one after the other, but without producing any effect upon the iris; his eyes were exactly an amaurotic person's, and all noticed their lack-lustre appearance. We were all now convinced that total insensibility of all the senses existed, and I ordered him to be placed on a mattrass on the floor, and not to be disturbed till I returned. It was now 1 o'clock, the process having commenced at 11 A. M.

I returned at 3 o'clock, and was vexed to find that he had awoke, and been carried back to the jail hospital. The native doctor of the jail had come in; and on hearing that the Sahibs could not awake the patient, he set about doing so, and succeeded by throwing water on his face, &c. I again went to Messrs. Russell and Money, and requested them to accompany me to the jail, to be present when he was interrogated regarding his reminiscences; and we put down a series of questions to be put to him, at once, and without explanation. We found him looking well, with a lively expression of face, and the following questions were put to him; his answers being taken down at the same time:—

"How do you feel?"

"Very well."

"Any pain in the throat, or elsewhere?"

"A little uneasiness in the throat, no pain anywhere else."

"What has happened to you to-day?"

"I went in the morning to the Imbarah Hospital, to get the water taken out of my scrotum."

"Was the water drawn off?"

"Yes."

"What do you remember after the operation?"

"I went to sleep soon after, and remember nothing else."

"Did you eat or drink after the operation?"

"I felt thirsty, but got nothing to drink till Kurreem Ali, the native doctor, awoke me."

"Did any body prick, or burn you?"

"No, no."

"Did you smell anything disagreeable?"

"No."

"Were you happy when asleep?"

"Very."

"Did you hear anything when you were asleep?"

"I heard voices, but did not understand them."

"Did you see any gentleman in the hospital but me?"

"No."

"Did you feel any pain in the scrotum after going to sleep?"

"I felt none till I awoke."

"Any pain in that part now?"

"A very little."

"How many motions have you had to-day?" (he was suffering from chronic diarrhœa.)

"Four, before going to the hospital, none since; belly is much easier than it has been for some time."

Having answered all these questions readily and frankly, he began to cry, thinking it was some kind of judicial investigation, I suppose.

"The above is an exact relation of what took place in our presence, and we are thoroughly convinced that there was a complete suspension of sensibility to external impressions of the most painful kind.

(Signed) F. W. RUSSELL.
D. J. MONEY.
BUDDEN CRUNDER CHOWDAREE,
Sub-Assistant Surgeon."

April 5th.—There is less than the usual inflammation, and he makes no complaint. I intend to operate on the other side in a few days, mesmerizing him first, if possible, and have invited many persons to be present.

Second Experiment.

April 6th.—11 o'clock, A. M. The inflammation has become high during last night; the part is hot, and excessively tender; the lightest touch causes great pain. Skin hot; pulse quick. I could not resist the temptation of satisfying myself still further, and relieve him at the same time. So, turning to the native doctors, I said that I would try the "Belatee Muntur" (the Europe charm,) and began the process as before; he lying in bed. In ten minutes the mesmeric haze (smoke he always calls it) was produced. After half an hour he still complained of the pain in the inflamed part, and could not bear its being touched; in three-quarters of an hour the coma was established, and I squeezed the inflamed part with no more effect than if it had been a bladder. Having business to attend to in Chandernagore, six miles off, I called, in passing, on the Rev. Mr. Fisher, and said that he might now satisfy himself by going to the hospital in my absence; and that, except mesmeric means, he was at liberty to use every possible means to awake him, or make him feel. Here I have the pleasure to introduce a report of the proceedings of Mr. Fisher and Mr. Money while I was at Chandernagore:—

"*To J. Esdaile, Esq.*

"My Dear Sir,—I beg to certify that I twice saw the native whom you had put into a mesmeric trance, or state of catalepsy, and from the successful application of different tests I have no hesitation in stating, should my statement add weight to your own testimony, or be of any service to the cause of the imperfectly known, and hitherto unfairly treated, science of Mesmerism, that the individual in question was in that state entirely insensible of pain, and that I believe, if you had cut his leg off, he would not have felt it. I saw, when I was in England, both publicly and in private, many cases of Mesmerism accompanied by unnatural and wonderful phenomena, without being convinced. But your case is one so free from all possibility of suspicion, that to have doubted it, one might as well have doubted his own existence. Yours truly,

"D. J. Money.

"*Hooghly, 9th April,* 1845."

"I have only to add to the above, that I was present upon the last occasion referred to by Mr. Money, and fully concur with him in thinking that the patient, during the Mesmeric trance, was totally insensible to pain. Indeed, all the senses appeared to be unnaturally suspended from any manifestation of their ordinary operations, and every available test was tried in vain. Dr. Esdaile upon this occasion was absent at Chandernagore, having previously put the patient into the trance.

"F. FISHER."

Returned to the hospital at 3 o'clock, and found him lying just as I had left him. Awoke him in a few minutes, by rapid transverse passes, blowing in his face, and giving water to drink. Is free of pain, and still desires to sleep; says his head turns.

Translation of a Report from Kurreem Ali Khan, native doctor, of what he saw and heard in the Jail Hospital, on the 6th April, 1845.

"At 11 o'clock, A. M., the patient, Madhab Kaura, was in a fever, and there was an acute pain in the scrotum. The worthy Dr. Sahib (may he ever prosper) came to the hospital, and began to do something to him. When the experiment was going on, Madhab was asked,—

"What do you see?"

"I cannot see clearly; something like smoke is before my eyes."

"Do you see the doors?"

"No, nothing but smoke."

"Do you see Dr. Sahib?"

"No, I see nobody, but perceive some one is talking near me."

"Is there any pain in your body?"

"Yes, breathing causes pain in the belly."

"Is there pain in the scrotum?"

"Yes, as acute as ever."

"How do you feel now?"

"I feel cold and sleepy."

After the Doctor Sahib had tried for nearly three-quarters of an hour, he fell into a deep sleep, and there seemed to be no pain in the scrotum; he slept so sound, that even the pricking of his body with a pin did not restore his senses, or awake him. Before, a touch of the scrotum was painful, but after he was asleep, even pricking it caused no pain whatever.

He continued in this state for three hours, when, the Dr. Sahib calling him aloud twice or thrice, he came to his senses, and opened his eyes. He asked for water, which he drank, and, feeling cold, covered himself."

Translation of a Report from Noboo, native doctor, of what he saw and heard in the Jail Hospital, on the 6th April, 1845.

"On the morning of the 6th of April, I went to the hospital, and found the body of Madhab Kaura hot and feverish, and he felt a great pain in the scrotum.

At 11 o'clock, Dr. Esdaile, the civil doctor, came and made some operations on the body: something I do not know. While the operation was going on, the patient was asked if he could see plainly, but said no. When asked if he could see any one, he answered, that he could see no one, but knew by the sounds that some people were there.

Again he was asked if he felt any pain; he said, that he felt a severe pain in the belly, on breathing, and also in the scrotum, and felt very cold. Soon afterwards he became senseless.

At 2 o'clock P. M. the Rev. Mr. Fisher and Mr. Money came to the hospital, and tried to bring him to his senses by pricking him with a pin, putting fire on his hand, and beating a gong in his ear, but all proved ineffectual."

I forgot to note down what these reports notice;—his complaining of feeling cold soon after the process began; and that when I left him the temperature of his body was natural.

On these two occasions, the effects were witnessed by all the patients and hangers-on in and about both hospitals.

April 7th.—Has had a good night, is a little feverish; pain in the scrotum much less. He now complains, for the first time, of pain in the places where he was pricked and burned.

This makes one ashamed of incredulity, and I will never put a patient to the "question" in this way again. It is only excusable for the first time, when we can hardly believe the evidence of our senses.

Third Experiment.

April 11th.—Took the sub-assistant surgeon with me to-day to the Jail Hospital, and desired him to watch the time taken to produce the different effects. There is still considerable pain in the side operated upon. Pulse regular, 60; skin warm. At 11 o'clock A. M. I seated him on the floor with his back against the wall; placed myself before him on a stool, and proceeded pretty much as before. The process, in one particular, was varied; I leaned my elbows upon my knees, placed my mouth over the back of my joined hands, and breathed along their upper surface; the points of my fingers being pointed steadily at his eyes, nose, and forehead, in succession. This seemed to be very effectual, and was done with the idea of concentrating the mesmeric influence of the whole body into one conductor. It was curious to observe that he had begun to think on the subject, and was observing the effects for himself, and testing his senses as we proceeded. After manipulating for a few minutes, he opened his eyes, looked sharply and minutely about him, and being asked if he saw quite well, he said, "Oh, yes." In a minute or two he repeated his inspection, and answered again, that he saw quite distinctly; in seven minutes he again looked about him, seemed surprised, and said he only saw "smoke."

In fifteen minutes he was pinched; and when asked if any one was pinching him, he replied that he could not tell, as I might now cut a piece out of his body without his feeling it. I now tried for an abnormal mental manifestation; certainly not expecting to be gratified. I asked,—"What will cure your complaint?"

"You know best."

"Has the Baboo any complaint?"

"How should I know?"

I understood this as a hint to attend to the business in hand, the body, and therefore proceeded to induce the mesmeric coma as quickly as possible; and succeeded in twenty minutes from the commencement. I then said to the sub-assistant surgeon that I would operate upon him in this state, if I could find some of the European gentlemen to be witnesses. On going to Chinsurah, two miles off. I fortunately found a considerable party, consisting of the Baron Law de Clapernou, Governor of Chandernagore, Mr. Russell, the judge, Mr. Wauchope, the magistrate, J. St. Pourcain, Esq., Mr. Clint, Principal of Hooghly College, and Mr. Clermont, head master of the Lower School; who all accompanied me back to the hospital. The man had fallen down, and was lying on his back. The large gong of the jail was brought, and struck violently within a few inches of his ear, with no effect. I then pierced the scrotum, and threw in the injection, without any one being sensible of the smallest movement in his face or body. His limbs were quite flexible; but on holding one of his legs in my hand for a few seconds, it gradually became quite rigid, and we could not bend it again; the same occurred in the other leg. The arms were supple, and lay in any position into which they were thrown; and when the fore-arm was bent upon the humerus, and then let go, it fell upwards, or downwards, instantly. But on placing my united fingers over the ends of his, the arm remained fixed at a right angle in the air, and swayed to and fro, according to my movements. The insensibility of the iris was also tested, and proved.

6 o'clock, P. M. Still sleeps; most complete relaxation of all the limbs now exists. The legs and arms can be tossed about in every direction, and where they fall there they lie. Being curious to ascertain the effect of the artificial state on the natural process of inflammation, I did not awake him, but saw that the part was as flaccid as when the water was just withdrawn.

April 12th.—He awoke at 12 o'clock last night, spontaneously. Recollects nothing after going to sleep; sees the water is gone, knows not how; supposes the Dr. Sahib did it. The testicle is considerably enlarged to-day; there is little pain, and it did not swell till after he awoke. He has had chronic diarrhœa for some time; four and five motions a day, but has had none since yesterday forenoon till this morning. Natural, artificial, and diseased actions have therefore been all equally arrested for the last thirteen hours; a practical fact of the utmost importance, which will not be lost sight of by myself, or others, I hope. What a blessed prospect this opens to sufferers who may be sensible to the Mesmeric influence! In time we may hope to discover who they are, by detecting the laws which regulate this power of Nature, and thereby save ourselves much trouble and disappointment. In the mean time let us accumulate *facts,* as the seed for a correct theory hereafter. Although I should never succeed again, I will in future think, speak, and write of Mesmerism as being as much a reality as the principle of gravitation, or the properties of opium. For, under all the circumstances, I cannot but consider these to be unexceptionable *facts;* and if I should not again be able to elicit them, it would not shake my belief in the existence of Mesmerism; I should only conclude that the failure arose from my ignorance of the conditions required by Nature, or from some personal disqualification. The rarity of the occurrence would not make it less a reality; and to deny a fact because it has been seldom witnessed, would be as reasonable as to doubt the existence of comets because they are rare appearances.

Great weight is very justly attached to *first experiments* in any new subject of investigation, for these are often a voluntary and unexpected evolution of the powers of nature; and when the results surprise the experimenter even, we feel confident that he only relates what he actually saw, and that he is not seduced, by previous theory and prepossession of mind, to interpret appearances in support of a foregone conclusion. In making these experiments, I was in the situation of a chemist, who has heard that a new elementary substance had been discovered by a certain process, and who thereupon sets his apparatus to work in the way prescribed, and is rewarded by obtaining the same results as the first discoverer.

Besides the general results, I noted in this case the following particulars as *facts,* which determined the course of my future proceedings.

I was sure that there could be no imagination at work in the matter.

That there was no consent between the parties.

No mental sympathy.

That the patient's eyes need not be open.

I therefore came to the conclusion, that in this instance, the influence must have been of a purely physical description, and on this supposition I conducted my subsequent experiments; with what success will be shortly seen.

CHAPTER III.

Mesmerism the same in India and in Europe.—Examples of Mesmeric Sleep.—Sealing of the Eyes.—Altered Sensibility.—Temporary Paralysis.—Muscular Rigidity.—Insensibility to Pain.—Exaltation of particular Organs.—Convulsions.—Delirium.—Injustice done to the Memory of the first Mesmerists.—Every available Evidence here given.—Imposture morally and physically impossible.—Mode of Proceeding.—Mesmeric and Non-Mesmeric Operations contrasted.—Physiological Demonstration of the Impossibility of Imposture.

HAVING, by the experiments described in the last chapter, satisfied myself of the existence of the Mesmeric power, I lost no time in applying it to practical purposes. The effects produced were nearly as various as the different persons acted upon, and corresponded perfectly with the appearances observed in Europe; and when the public see the same effects following like causes on the banks of the Thames, and the Seine, the Rhine, and the Hooghly; I presume it will conclude, that the same agent is at work, provided the same evidence, in support of matters of fact, is received for hot and cold climates, and it is not supposed that the truth is affected by degrees of latitude. In a late number of the "British and Foreign Medical Review," the reviewer gives a summary of the Mesmeric symptoms as known to himself, and recorded by various writers on Mesmerism, and acknowledges a perfect accord in all the accounts of the bodily phenomena. The following extract will place these appearances succinctly before my readers, and I beg them to compare my account of Mesmerism in Bengal with this statement of its effects in Europe, and then say whether the identity of the thing in the east and west is not established:—

"Sometimes, however, there is said to supervene a state of coma; at others, exaltation, depression, or some anomalous modification of sensibility; and occasionally, a state somewhat approaching to that of reverie, wherein the individual, although conscious, feels incapable of independent exertion, and spell-bound, as it were, to a particular train of thought or feeling. The occurrence of convulsive action, and of muscular rigidity, is described as taking place in some cases to a greater or less extent. These results are said to constitute the *simpler phenomena* of Mesmerism. We shall illustrate them by some extracts from accredited writers upon the subject.

"In this peculiar state of sleep, the surface of the body is sometimes acutely sensible, but more frequently the sense of feeling is absolutely annihilated. The jaws are firmly locked, and resist every effort to wrench them open; the joints are often rigid, and the limbs inflexible; and not only is the sense of feeling, but the senses of smell, hearing, and sight also, are so deadened to all external impressions, that no pungent odour, loud report, or glare of light, can excite them in the slightest degree. The body may be pricked, pinched, lacerated, or burnt; fumes of concentrated liquid ammonia may be passed up the nostrils; the loudest reports suddenly made close upon the ear; dazzling and intense light may be thrown upon the pupil of the eye; yet so profound is the physical state of lethargy, that the sleeper will remain undisturbed and insensible to tortures, which in the waking state, would be intolerable."—(*Dupotet,* p. 36.)

The above concise sketch corresponds very closely with what is laid down in other works of Mesmeric repute. A few brief quotations, exhibiting this correspondence, we subjoin. The first we take from Deleuze's Practical Instructions, wherein he states that "the magnetised feels the necessity of closing the eyes; his eyes are so sealed that he cannot open them; he experiences a calm, a feeling of comfort; he becomes drowsy; he is put to sleep."—Teste, another writer of distinction, speaking of the physical insensibility, says, "it exists, not only in the skin, but in the subcutaneous tissues, in the muscles, and even in the nervous ramifications." Dr. Passavant of Frankfort, an author often referred to, avers as follows: "As an especial effect of the power of animal magnetism, results the magnetic sleep. This is mostly deeper than ordinary sleep, the mediation of the senses is yet more decidedly suspended. The sensibility can so have vanished in a moment, that the loudest sound, the brightest light, even bodily injuries, are not perceived in this sleep." Indeed, all the authorities seem to coincide very much in their accounts, and, this we say, after referring to Chenevix, Elliotson, Townshend, Gauthier, Foissac, and others."

I shall now present to the reader illustrations of all the singular states of the system described above, and drawn from my practice here.

Mesmeric Sleep.—This simulates, perfectly, sound natural sleep, and is more refreshing, even if it has been resorted to for soothing pain, or disturbance of the system, and can be had recourse to when it would be improper or useless to administer common narcotics;—over which it has the advantage of not inducing a disagreeable constitutional derangement, after the specific influence has ceased. The restorative powers of mesmeric sleep seem to depend upon an actual infusion of nervous vigour into the body, and, when induced as a remedial agent, this may account for its superiority over common sleep.

April 7th.—Janokee-Sing, a hardy looking peon; the whole of the scrotum is sloughing, from the application of some acrid leaves, and the pain is most intense.

April 15th.—The whole scrotum has sloughed off; has not slept since coming to hospital. The compounder, a healthy, intelligent Hindoo, succeeded in putting him to sleep to-day, in half an hour. He awoke when pinched, or called upon by name, but instantly fell asleep again.

April 16th.—Has slept, almost without interruption, from 11 o'clock A. M. yesterday till 7 o'clock this morning, the only sleep he has had since he was burned.

April 19th.—He has been mesmerised daily, and sleeps the greater part of his time; to mesmerise him, becomes more easy every day;—and a few minutes now suffice to overcome him.

April 20th.—Kowsoalla; aged forty, a peasant woman. I subdued her to-day, for the first time, in ten minutes; she awoke when called upon, but, in a second, fell asleep again. The limbs are quite loose, but when I let them remain for a moment in any new position, they become rigid, and require to be dragged into a new attitude; the muscles yield precisely like lead, without a vestige of re-action, when the bending force is removed.

April 25th.—She can now be mesmerised in a minute.

May 3rd.—Bissumber Chowdry: has had retention of urine for three days; the bladder is prominent at the navel, and no instrument can be introduced. Ordered to lie in the easiest posture, and to be put to sleep, if possible.

May 4th.—He slept for two hours yesterday, and voided his urine freely, when he awoke.

May 4th.—Deenoo, a prisoner; convalescent from cholera, is tormented with incessant hiccough for the last twenty-four hours.

Opii Grs. ii.
Confect. Arom. Grs. x.

If this does not check it, a blister to be applied over the diaphragm.

May 5th.—No better—To be mesmerised. I returned after three hours, and found him asleep—awoke him: has no hiccough.

May 11th.—No return of the hiccough.

Sealing of the eyes.—The quivering of the eyelids, and their subsequent spasmodic closure, is one of the most specific mesmeric symptoms.

June 27th.—The woman Alunga complains of considerable pain from the extension of her arm yesterday, and the nerve at the elbow is very tender. I passed my fingers along the course of the nerve for a few minutes, which removed the pain; I then held my fingers before her eyes, and in a few seconds she fell into my arms quite insensible. I soon after awoke her, and she sat up conversing with us as usual, but could not possibly open her eyes; when ordered to do so, she was obliged to pull the eyelids asunder with her fingers; but they would not remain open, and the difficulty was only removed by my rubbing, and blowing in her eyes. I have shown this peculiarity, in numerous cases, to great numbers of persons.

Altered sensibility.—Rajah ——, an intelligent Hindoo gentleman, who has received an English education, and speaks our language perfectly well, wished to be operated on for hydrocele, while in the mesmeric trance. After half an hour's manipulating, I extended his arm, and it took a fix in any position I put it: it was put perpendicular into the air, and remained motionless for ten minutes; on depressing it again, it bent like lead, in the true cataleptic fashion. Having replaced his arm at his side, I began to open his dress, when he awoke with a violent start, and instantly said that he had no feeling in his arm; that it was very cold, which we all felt, and on putting a thermometer into his hand, we found it to be two degrees colder than the other. He remembered my raising his arm, and felt me let go my hold of his thumb, but what became of his arm after that, he could not tell—he imagined it was lost. Having lately felt the sensation of galvanism, he said, that he felt slight shocks in his skin during the process, exactly like what he had experienced from galvanism. I have observed this in other patients.

Temporary paralysis of muscles.—Madub, a shopkeeper. This man was operated on for hydrocele, when in the trance, without feeling it, and ever since has been very easily affected; I have, therefore, made him the subject of several experiments. In a minute or two, his eyelids begin to quiver, then slowly close, opening heavily at short intervals, till at last they remain closed altogether. If at this stage he is ordered to open his eyes, the effort to do so only strains the eyelids, which appear to be glued together, and he says it is impossible to separate them. Being desired to help himself with his fingers, he rubs his eyes violently, and then forcibly separates the eye-lids, when nothing but the white of the eye is seen; the cornea being turned up to the roof of the orbit. While rubbing his eyes, I sometimes seize his hands and extend his arms horizontally on either side; the arms become fixed in a moment, and when desired to apply his hands to his eyes now, he says that he cannot, that he does not know where his arms are. If I blow on one arm, or impel a current of air against it by fanning, the rigidity disappears, and he uses his arm as desired, but the other continues catalepsed and useless, till relieved in the same way. When I urge him to use both arms, he says he has only one, and on being desired to seek for the other, he passes the flexible arm across his body, and gropes at the other side for it, but soon gives up the search, saying, it is not there: being desired to look for it higher up, he carries his hand up the opposite side till he reaches the catalepsed arm, and tries in vain to depress it; the arm remains horizontally extended, and resists all his efforts.

Muscular rigidity.—Is usually attendant on mesmeric coma, of which numerous instances will be given, when treating of the medical part of the subject. My first patient, by repeated experiments, became excessively sensitive, and affords a good specimen of mesmeric catalepsy.

May 13th.—Madub Kaura; this man can be catalepsed in less than a minute; and the effects are passing strange. If, when he is standing, I point my fingers at him for a few seconds, his eyelids immediately droop, his arms fall by their mere weight to his sides; his whole body begins to tremble, owing to the incipient loss of command over the muscular system; and, if not supported, he would fall down in a heap. But give him a moment's support, and he becomes as rigid as a statue, and if the centre of gravity is well poised he will remain in any posture he is put into, and that for a longer time than I have waited to see. The muscles must be dragged out of the fixed position they have assumed, and allowed a moment to contract in a new attitude, out of the perpendicular; for if suddenly pushed, he goes down, head foremost, like a statue from its pedestal, and his life is endangered.

However inconvenient, or grotesque, the position may be, he is equally well satisfied, and continues to sleep, quite comfortably, with his heels behind his neck; and if his forehead is placed against the wall at an acute angle, he remains sticking out from it, like a buttress, longer than I have ascertained.

Insensibility to pain.—This will be copiously illustrated in my numerous surgical operations.

Somnambulism.—Will have a chapter to itself, and need not be now introduced.

Exaltation of particular organs,—convulsions,—delirium.—Instances of all these will occur in the course of this work, and be found to correspond with the irregularities observed in Europe; so that the general rule, and its exceptions, will be recognised to be the same in the eastern and the western hemispheres; thereby proving the universality of the truths declared by many honest and independent men, during the last sixty years, and for propounding which they were laughed at, and scorned.

Apart from the personal gratification of being admitted to see the secret processes of nature's workshop, and the advantages of being able to imitate her processes, for the alleviation and removal of human suffering; it will be a great satisfaction to me, if any evidence and labours should assist in raising the dishonoured dead into the public consideration and respect, due to them as benefactors of mankind, and in exciting a regret that wisdom called so long in the streets, without any one regarding her.

I now know (and I deplore my long ignorance) that the battle was fought, and won, before I was born, by the truthful and benevolent Puysegur, Deleuze, and their companions, and that I, under the tropics, am only again demonstrating what they, on the banks of the Seine, had long ago established. The people of the continent have been familiar with both the good and evil of Mesmerism for the last thirty years, while we in England are only now giving an unwilling ear to the expounders of a law of nature, which is as much a part of the human constitution as the processes of thought and digestion. It is to be hoped that, on this subject, our neighbours will no longer have reason to reproach our insular ignorance and presumption, and that if Mesmerism is rejected by the English public, it will be after study and experiment, and not from prejudice and passion.

Knowing the new and wonderful nature of the subject, and that the public was ill prepared to receive the naked truth on individual testimony, I have called in all the available evidence on the spot; and the facts related by me will be found to be vouched for by disinterested, honourable, and intelligent gentlemen, both residents and strangers; and if there is not a cloud of European witnesses, it is simply because no more exist in this neighbourhood. I would have preferred the plain of Calcutta for my theatre, and all the inhabitants for spectators, if it had been possible. All I have done, or may hereafter do, has been done, and shall be done, in open day, and every case related has had from half a dozen to hundreds of witnesses. The patients are on the spot, or can easily be found, and a host of eye-witnesses are ready for any one who may take the trouble to investigate the matter on the spot.

Taking these general circumstances into account, I might leave the cases to be adduced to speak for themselves, but I hope to be excused for pointing out some particulars which will, I trust, demonstrate that imposture, in the generality of my cases, is morally and physically impossible.

It is *morally* impossible that I could have taught my patients what I did not know; for I knew not the existence of the diversified symptoms they exhibited, till, day by day, I became a witness of their unexpected occurrence. I had never read a Mesmeric book, when I made my first experiment; and having succeeded in getting nature to speak, I determined to listen only to her for some time, and for months purposely refrained from reading on the subject, in order that my senses might not be predisposed to see things in any particular light, and that my judgment might be left unbiased by the opinions of others. My reason did not teach me to expect what was presented to my senses; but was gradually instructed by what I saw and did: and all that I know about Mesmerism has been acquired by reading the book of nature, without guide or interpreter. If I was ignorant of the subject, the peasants and coolies of Bengal must have been equally so, I presume. No rumour had gone abroad regarding the existence of such a power; Mesmerism had not become the village talk in Bengal, so as to enable some clever rogue to exhibit the phenomena of which he had heard:—there was no type to imitate, therefore imitation, in the first instance, was impossible. Be it observed also, that the cases did not happen among people in hospitals at the same time, but arose, day by day, among patients newly arrived from different parts of the country. The routine followed is this. A person presents himself before me for the first time, and I see he has a disease requiring an operation for its removal; he is desired to go into another room (which is dark,) and repose himself after his journey, not a word being said about an operation, as this would cause a mental excitement, destructive to the mesmeric influence. One of my assistants follows him; seats himself (if unperceived, so much the better,) at the head of the bed; and by using the process to be hereafter described, often reduces the patient to a state of coma by the end of my visit: I then do what is necessary, whether it be to take off, or straighten a limb, without his knowledge or consent. Now, supposing these poor ignorant people to be impostors, whence comes their intimate knowledge of the mesmeric phenomena, from the quivering of an eye-lid onwards to insensibility to the most cruel tortures? If they are not what they seem to be, then are they heaven-born impostors, or have had supernatural instruction,—on earth they could not have learned it.

It may be said, that it is the taste of the coolies of Bengal to have themselves cut to pieces, and to have corrosive acids, and red-hot pokers applied to their sores, without showing a sign of life; or that, knowing my hobby, they come from all quarters to be silently tormented, in order to please my Honour. Or we may be told, that the passive endurance of pain is no sign of the absence of it, for the North American invites his enemy to tear him at the stake, and the Indian Fuqueer voluntarily torments himself.

To do justice to this ingenious hypothesis, I shall present the reader with some examples of the way in which pain is borne by my patients, in the mesmeric and non-mesmeric condition of the body.

June 12th.—Lokee, a peasant woman, aged 60, has a tumour on the calf of the leg of nine years' standing; it is full of deep ulcerations and maggots. I tried to subdue her yesterday, but the pain did not allow her to get beyond common sleep. To-day, after much trouble, first by one person, and then another, she was entranced, and I cut out the tumour in the presence of Captain Elder, without her feeling it, and we left her sleeping.

June 13th.—She awoke three hours after the operation; felt no pain on waking, and asked me to-day, who cut off the tumour?

Oct. 24th.—The woman Lokee has come back to hospital, with a return of the tumour, cut out in June last, to be mesmerised.

Oct. 27th.—She has been mesmerised daily, for two hours, but without effect. I therefore operated on her to-day, as we could spare no more time for her, others requiring equal attention. The poor old woman screamed miserably the whole time, crying, that I was murdering her; and she continued in the greatest pain for hours afterwards.

If the old woman shammed insensibility on the first occasion, why did she not do so on the second? She had had practice; every facility and encouragement were given her, and she knew what was wanted of her, and yet would not pretend to be asleep!

This perverse and inconsistent conduct appears to me to be easily accounted for, from the very fact of her being aware of what was wanted and intended to be done; her anxiety to go to sleep neutralised her good intentions:—excitement of mind being destructive of the mesmeric influence for the production of coma.

August 13th.—Dr. Finch freely applied muriatic acid (such as is furnished by the Company's dispensary) to a sore, covering all the right temple of the woman Gendo (who was mesmerised, in his presence, by one of my assistants,) without her showing the smallest degree of consciousness; and it was with great difficulty I awoke her, after he had failed to do so. During the burning with the acid, her pulse fell from 88° to 80°, and her respiration, which was quite natural before she was mesmerised, became entirely diaphragmatic, and abdominal; the voluntary and semi-voluntary muscles of the chest being completely paralysed.

August 18th.—Dr. Bedford to-day asked permission to apply the acid to the woman Gendo's sore, when she was awake; and though I thought this most irrational scepticism (he having witnessed Dr. Finch's experiment) I consented, in order that it might not be said that I interfered to save my phenomena. He accordingly wetted the end of the glass stopper with the acid, and touched the sore with it, and the woman, for a few seconds, did not show any signs of acute pain. There could be no doubt about it, she was found out! The arch deceiver, having set a snare and delusion for me, was now laughing at my beard; and I was not relieved from my thick-coming fancies by Dr. B. kindly suggesting, "that she was probably a very insensible person naturally." I was soon roused from my trance of bewilderment, however, by hearing the woman cry out, that "we had put pepper to her head!" and she sat up, showing signs of great pain; immediately after, she declared "her head was on fire," and got out of bed, walking about distractedly in great agony. I ordered her head to be bathed, and, as the best anodyne, threw her into the trance: the sore being surrounded by tubercles, which retarded its healing, I took the opportunity to pare them off; and to this she was perfectly indifferent. In half an hour, I awoke her with much difficulty, in order that Dr. B. might hear her first words, which were, that she knew nothing about what we were talking of, having even forgotten the burning; an invasion of the waking by the sleeping state, which will be seen in another patient, when Mrs. Clermont's case is given. So that if Mesmerism did not protect this old woman, we have the curious fact of muriatic acid, applied in large quantities to a raw surface by Dr. Finch, acting as a direct anodyne and narcotic, calming at the same time the circulation, and revolutionising the respiration, while a drop in the hands of Dr. Bedford causes the greatest suffering and general excitement!—"*Non nobis tantas componere lites.*"

Oct. 10th.—Beppo Dass, a prisoner, was entranced to-day; in the presence of Dr. Roer, Mr. Bradbury, Major Riddell, Mr. Higgins, Mr. Muller, Mr. Graves, Messrs, Savigny, Mr. Bartlett; and I operated on him for hydrocele. The injection was thrown in without his showing a vestige of feeling, and his arm, which I had placed in the air, on purpose, at the commencement, never moved, and had to be taken down after the operation; this was the second operation performed on the man during the last fortnight; and on both occasions he slept for two hours afterwards, knew nothing of what had happened on waking, and felt no pain till the artificial inflammation commenced at 9 o'clock at night; the operation having been performed at noon. This has been called a painless operation.

"They laugh at scars who never felt a wound,"

and I shall therefore transcribe a passage from a friend's letter, written shortly after the publication of my first case.

"When I was first operated on, some years ago, for hydrocele, and the injection was thrown up, the pain was like a coir rope, round my loins, being pulled at each end by some persons as hard as they could; and the perspiration ran down my head as if some one was sprinkling water on my hair; so this is what you have laid dormant by your Mesmerism."

But it is for the sequel of this case, that I here quote it, and in order to show the man's behaviour in his natural and artificial states. On the day after the operation, the inflammation is usually high, and from the sensitive nature of the parts, pressure is excessively painful. Now, on both occasions, I have requested numerous gentlemen to press the part, and ascertain if it was *really* painful: "a question not to be asked," was always their reply. The man was then entranced, and the experiment repeated by the same persons, when he allowed the part to be pressed as if it was a bottle:—he was then awakened, and on being now pressed, showed all the signs of instant and acute pain.

The cases above cited, along with, if I may use the expression, very numerous *painless severe* surgical operations, might be safely adduced as demonstrations of the physical impossibility of imposture; but I shall now submit to the physiologist a series of facts which, to him, will be more convincing than all the cutting, tearing, and lacerating we can invent. For although we may pretty certainly conclude, that men will not exhibit insensibility to torture, without some adequate object to be gained, yet the incentive may escape our observation, or be unintelligible to us. It is, therefore, desirable to discover something which it was *impossible* for a man in a natural condition to do, under the influence of any passion, or under the temptation of the highest bribe. To perform the following feats, will, I imagine, be found above the power of the most accomplished impostor: to keep the pupils dilated, without the use of drugs, in passing from darkness into sunshine,—to lower the pulse at pleasure,—to breathe only by the diaphragm, for hours, and diminish the temperature of the body, at will. The dilation and insensibility of the pupil are recorded in my first case, and have since been frequently seen.

June 11th.—Kaloo, a Fuqueer, has an excrescence, larger than a man's fist, at the end of his penis, and the body of the organ is also much enlarged. I entranced him in a few minutes, on the first trial, and in the presence of Major Riddell, Captain Anderson, Mr. Bennett, and Mr. Jackson, dissected out the organ, but was obliged to sacrifice the glans, as it was a cartilaginous degeneration of all the structures of the part:—the man did not awake till I was amputating the organ, after a long dissection. Wonderful to say, he relapsed into the trance again in a few minutes, and remained for twenty minutes, quite rigid, and insensible, with his eyes wide open, and the pupils dilated, in a full noonday light, to which they were wholly insensible. This is not the only instance in which the eyes have been wide open during the trance, and would not remain shut when I closed them, showing, I conceive, the absolute extinction of muscular power. In most cases the muscles of the eyeball continue to act involuntarily, after the rest of the muscular system has gone to rest, and on opening the eyelids, the ball of the eye is seen rolling round the orbit, like an agitated magnetic needle. Under the most intense degree of the influence, the msucles of the eye, and iris, also lose their contractibility, and the eye becomes as motionless and insensible to light as that of a dead man. That the second trance was not a faint, we all satisfied ourselves, not only from the general rigidity of the body, but from the regular *natural pulse.*

Sept. 17th.—In the presence of the Reverend Mr. Fisher and Dr. Heathcote, I to-day operated for cataract on a man while in the mesmeric trance. The pupil was so much dilated that Dr. H. asked if belladonna had been applied? After depressing the lens, and withdrawing the needle, the lens rose again, and such was the continued dilation of the pupil, that it passed into the anterior chamber, and came in contact with the cornea; the man being insensible all the time.

Sept. 18th.—To-day, in the presence of the Reverend Mr. Bradbury, I entranced a man for the first time, in the hope of subduing an inflammation of one eye, by removing all pain and irritation, and thereby allowing the restorative powers of nature to act undisturbed; he was entranced sitting on a stool, in order to lessen the flow of blood to the head. We counted his pulse beforehand; it was 100 in the minute; respiration 20; thoracic movement natural; temperature higher than usual. After 20 minutes, his pulse had sunk to 70, his respiration to 18, and, by comparing his chest with that of a man lying alongside of him, we ascertained that there was *not a vestige of thoracic movement.* All above the diphragm was as fixed as the trunk of a statue, and the temperature of his body had become lower than natural.

If these tests are not considered an "*experimentum crucis,*" I am at a loss to imagine what will be reckoned more satisfactory by the human physiologist. It appears to me, that when we see the *involuntary* organs of the body revolutionised, it is absurd to attribute it to the effect of the *will.*

CHAPTER IV.

Somnambulism.—Definition.—Singular Introduction to it.—Suspected Child-Stealing by its Means.—First Experiment in making a Somnambulist.—Trial of Mesmeric Skill in a Court of Justice.—Men stolen out of Court.—Truth of Mesmerism publicly proved.—Natural Sleep, and its Varieties, can be imitated by Artificial Means.—Mesmeric Sleep.—Mesmeric Day-mare.—Mesmeric Sleep-walking.—Mesmeric Sleep-waking.—Mesmeric Dreaming.—How to make Somnambulists.—Imitative Stage of Somnambulism.—Communicative Stage of Somnambulism.—Mesmeric Catalepsy.—Mesmeric Coma.—Natural Clairvoyance.—Mesmeric Clairvoyance.—Nature of the Mesmeric Power.—Illustrative Examples.

BEFORE submitting to the reader the results of my observations on somnambulism, I beg leave to prefix the following summary of the appearances recognised as distinctive of the somnambulistic state in Europe. It is given in the British and Foreign Medical Review, already quoted:—"Somnambulism is a condition in which certain senses and faculties are suppressed, or rendered thoroughly impassive, whilst others prevail in most unwonted exaltation; in which an individual, though asleep, feels and acts most energetically, holding an anomalous species of communication with the external world, awake to objects of attention, and most profoundly torpid to things at the time indifferent; a condition respecting which, most commonly, the patient on awaking retains no recollection; but, on any relapse into which a train of thought and feeling related to, and associated with, the antecedent paroxysm, will very often be developed."

I intended to have reserved this branch of the subject till I had examined it in all its purely medical bearings; but I was forced, by most extraordinary circumstances, to enter prematurely into this difficult and obscure field of experiment, in order to enable me to give my evidence in a court of justice; and in describing my experiments, I hope it will be borne in mind, that I had never seen a somnambulist, or thought of making one, up to this date. My first essay was as extemporaneous and accidental as the production of mesmeric coma, on the first occasion I tried to mesmerise:—the facts are simply these.

June 17th.—About a fortnight ago, I was driving through Hooghly Bazaar, and saw a crowd collected before the police office. On asking what was the matter, I was told that a man had been apprehended in the act of stealing a boy, and that the parties were inside the guard-house. Upon hearing this, I entered the house, and found a boy of ten or twelve years old, sitting on the lap of a man who was said to have rescued him. The boy was half stupid, and one of his eyes was swollen; I therefore ordered him to be taken to the hospital. The culprit was then shown to me. He said he was a barber; and a bundle containing his instruments of trade, was produced; this I carefully examined, but only found the usual barber's tools. The boy soon recovered his senses, and told me, readily and consistently, the following tale, which I again heard him repeat before the magistrate, in a different sequence, but without a tittle of variation. He said, that early in the morning he went into a field close to a house, and that shortly after, a strange man left the road, and came up to him: as soon as he was near him, he began to mutter charms, and then took hold of his hand; very soon after, he passed his hand across his eyes, and that thereupon he lost his senses, and only recollected that the man led him away, but without force, and that he felt compelled to follow him. When he came to his senses, it was at the gate of Chandernagore, two miles from where he had met the man; and this was all he had to say. He had not eaten, drunk, or smoked, in company with the man; and his master and friends all said he was a clever, well-behaved boy, and had never been known to have fits, or walk in his sleep. I then examined the man who was said to have rescued him: his evidence was to this effect; that on the morning in question, he saw the boy, whom he knew very well, following a strange man; that he stopped him, and asked what he was doing there? The boy made no answer, and appeared to be idiotic: upon seeing this, he became alarmed, brought water to throw on his face, and used other means to revive him; in which he at last succeeded. On again questioning him, he said that he did not know why he was there; that he was obliged to follow that man, though he did not know him, and after saying this, he fell down, and bruised his eye on the ground. In the mean time, the man was making off, but was apprehended, and brought to Hooghly. I then called in the barber; and this was his story: he met the boy on the road crying and looking stupid, and on asking him what ailed him he said that he had lost his way. Upon hearing this, he desired the boy to accompany him to the police station, and that a policeman would take him home. The strange nature of the transaction, whichever side was true, strongly arrested my attention, and the trade of the man roused my suspicions; as I had heard that barbers in this country, while performing their tedious processes, could put people to sleep; and reports are rife, all over the country, of people having been obliged to follow persons who had charmed them; and the victims are said to be usually women. The barbers, all over the world, are a shrewd, observing race; their occupation brings them into close contact with the surfaces most sensitive to the mesmeric influence; and they are, therefore, very likely to have become possessed of the secret of Mesmerism at an early period, and perhaps it has descended to them as a mystery of their craft. I could only see two roads out of the dilemma: it was either a case of natural, or artificial somnambulism; and if the latter, how could it be brought about unless by Mesmerism? As accident had made me a witness in the case, I anticipated that I should be called upon to speak as to the possibility of such a mode of abduction; and as I was completely ignorant of the subject, I determined to make experiments, to satisfy myself. I thought it probable, that if this could be done by Mesmerism, I should perhaps be able to imitate it, as the greater power includes the less; and that I had only to stop short in the progress to insensibility, in order to produce like effects, if obtainable by this means.

I therefore repaired to the Jail Hospital, and mesmerised a man; in whom I had subdued inflammation of the eye, by entrancing him several times; but only went to the extent of inducing the cataleptic tendency, and leaving him the power of moving and hearing, but very imperfectly. At this point, I led him away, and then letting him go, he stalked to the other end of the enclosure, till brought up by the wall; being turned, he walked in a straight line till some obstacle obstructed him, and then stood helplessly still. If allowed to stand motionless for some minutes, the trance deepened, and he became insensible to sounds; by blowing in his eyes, and addressing him all the time, he revived, and repeated after me, with great exactness, both English and Hindostanee; on awakening him, he had no recollection of any part of his proceedings, and said that he had never stirred from the spot, although he was at the opposite end of the enclosure from where we commenced. Being summoned to the Magistrate's Court as a witness, I was asked, "if I thought it practicable to carry off a person in the way described in the evidence?" I replied, that "I thought it possible, because I had just done something very like it, by making a prisoner follow me round the hospital enclosure, without his knowing it." The magistrate committed the case; but when it came to be tried before the judge, it was found to be utterly impossible to convey even a glimpse of my meaning in the minds of the native law officers who had to try the case; and the judge therefore asked me if I had any objection to show the Moulavies in court that it was possible for one person to make another follow him involuntarily, as I said. I answered, that I was willing to make the experiment, but would engage to do nothing: if he would order three men, whom I named, to be sent for to Court, I would try what could be done,—the men to be kept in total ignorance of our intentions.

In a day or two after, I was requested to attend the judge's court, which was crowded with Europeans and natives. Nazir Mahomed was brought in, and placed at the bar: I mesmerised him in a few minutes, and led him, with his arms catalepsed, out of the court, and set him walking down the road for some distance, making his arms rigid in any position, as long as I pleased. I then replaced him at the bar, where the judge and Moulavies all addressed him, without his paying any attention to them; and they were obliged to ask me to awake him. This I did, and on being asked from the bench, if he had left the room since he first entered it, he confidently answered, "No." While they were speaking to him in front, I approached, unperceived, behind, and entranced him on the spot, in the act of speaking. The words died on his lips, and he became insensible to all voices that addressed him; he was again awoke by blowing in his eyes. Madub was put in the dock, and he did not see me on entering. The judge and Moulavies engaged him in conversation, and while he was speaking with animation and intelligence, I catalepsed him from behind, while in the usual praying attitude of a prisoner at the bar, and, in a moment, he ceased to speak or hear: I was told by those in front, that his lips moved as if in the act of speaking, after he ceased to be heard. He was so deeply affected that all motive power was nearly extinguished, and I had to push him from behind with my finger, to make him walk: he walked a few yards with difficulty, and then becoming suddenly rigid from head to foot, a slight push sent him down headlong upon the floor, in a most alarming manner: the fit of rigidity was so instantaneous that I was not aware of it. He was revived with some difficulty, and fortunately was not injured by his fall.

Sooroop Chund was next brought in, and, as I had not seen him for a month, I began asking him about his health, &c., mesmerising him all the time. In a few minutes, he ceased to answer, and I took him out of the dock, turned him round like a teetotum, his arms rigidly fixed all the time, and then restored him to his former place in a state of complete insensibility; no one could make him hear, or show the slightest sign of life. When I blew in his eyes, he instantly recovered his senses, and declared he had never left the spot.

Whether the barber stole the boy mesmerically or not, I will not pretend to decide, but it gave me an opportunity of proving, in the most public manner, that the thing could be done, and no one has ventured to deny publicly that I stole the men; and, with the facilities of a native barber, I could almost engage to steal a man, woman, or child, daily. From the moment that I witnessed the extreme degrees of Mesmerism, I became deeply impressed with a conviction of its power for evil as well as good; and I have driven it thus far, in the hope of rousing the public mind to a sense of the dangers, as well as benefits, that may be expected from it; and I trust the day is not distant, when public opinion will strongly condemn all those who practise the art, except for philosophic and medical purposes.

That the barber was in illegal possession of the boy's person, however obtained, was so clear, that he was sentenced to nine years' imprisonment, and labour in irons; and the sentence was confirmed by the superior court. But the government called for the proceedings, and thinking, I suppose, that the mesmeric experiments had made too deep an impression on the mind of the court, graciously pardoned the barber.

When puzzled by the unexpected exhibition of new and wonderful bodily, or mental phenomena, instead of solving our difficulties by denying the existence of the phenomena, or dismissing them contemptuously as the offspring of deception, or delusion, we shall do much better, and generally be nearer the truth, if we suspect that we have overlooked some power of the human constitution, and resolve diligently to betake ourselves to the study of the nature of the new agent. Like the careless knitter, we find, at the end of our work, that some stitches have been dropped, and that we must recommence our work *de novo.* By a comparison of the effects of natural and mesmeric sleep on the human system, it will be seen, I think, that they only differ in degree, and in the greater command we have over the artificial than the natural state of sleep; and I feel disposed to think that extreme conditions of the nervous system, its exhaustion or repletion, and the irregular distribution of the nervous secretions, produce the same effects on the bodily and mental organs in normal and abnormal sleep.

I shall attempt to exemplify this, by instituting a comparison between natural sleep and its diseased varieties, and the mesmeric phenomena; from which it will be apparent that most of the latter exist in the routine of life, and that the novelty consists in our being able to produce and vary them, at will, by a new direction of the nervous energy.

Common Sleep.—In this condition of the system there is an absolute repose of body and mind; at least, there is no consciousness of movement in either, on awaking.

Mesmeric Sleep exactly resembles common sleep, with added restorative and curative power, of which the following cases are examples.

July 8th.—Geereah, a Hindoo girl; aged 10: is suffering from suppression of urine for two days, in consequence of violence done to the perineum, by which the recto-vaginal septum has been destroyed: the bladder extends up to the navel, and no instrument can be passed, owing to the painful condition of the parts. I mesmerised her for half an hour, after which she slept an hour, and on waking voided her urine freely; all disagreeable symptoms immediately disappeared, and she was cured without a dose of medicine.

July 10th.—Oboychurn Roy, a Hindoo land-owner: had his left arm struck off, twelve days ago, in defending his house against a gang of *dacoits.* There are two white rings on his arm, made by ligatures applied to staunch the blood; and it is wonderful that mortification has not been produced. Several pieces of bone required to be removed, and this gave him great pain: he was mesmerised, locally, with great relief, and afterwards generally: he dropped asleep in half an hour, and slept the whole of that night; the only sleep he had had since the infliction of the injury.

2. *Night-mare.*—If the brain is disagreeably affected by internal physical impressions, such as an unequal distribution of

blood, or nervous energy, then a confused train of painful images take possession of the mind, which is filled with causeless fears and shadowy horrors; and the sleeper struggles helplessly to shake off the incubus that oppresses him.

Mesmeric day-mare.—This very much resembles *night-mare,* but with a greater tendency to walk and talk, and appears to depend upon the irregular distribution of the nervous power, and the consequent derangement of the respiration and circulation. This is so alarming an effect of Mesmerism, that I do not envy the amateur who may produce it.

July 4th.—Bunnoo, a Hindoo girl; aged 15. She sprained her ankle, ten days ago, by a fall: the foot, ankle, and half the leg, are much swollen, infiltrated, and very painful. I mesmerised her for an hour, but she only slept for a few minutes, and little relief was given.

July 5th.—She was again mesmerised to-day, and in ten minutes she became much agitated; her chest was convulsed, and she showed all the signs of a violent attack of hysteria. The convulsions were soothed in a short time, by generalising the mesmeric influence, and then she became delirious, crying out, that there was a man before her with great eyes, and desiring him to be taken away. Her eyes were wide open, but she said I was a Bengalee; thought she was in her own house, and did not know her own, or her mother's name, who was standing by her. I placed her mother before her, whom she took for a man, and ordered away, covering him with the choicest flowers of Bengalee abuse. She was sitting up, and carefully protecting her leg all this time, answering all my questions about *it* quite clearly. As it was not in a comfortable position, I desired her to place it to her liking, as she would not allow it to be touched: this she did, and said it was now right. I then asked, if she would go to sleep: she answered "yes;" upon which I pointed my fingers at her eyes, and she fell back as if shot, and went into the trance.

The leg could now be freely pressed all over, without disturbing her, and I made my assistants apply their hands to it, to show them that the heat had also disappeared; the inflamed parts were now cooler than our hands.

This was not a case in which the mesmeric trance could rapidly subdue inflammation; it was of too long standing, and the ligaments had been too much injured, but local manipulations gave great relief, and induced sleep even.

Sleep-walking.—Sometimes from irritability of the muscular system, there is a craving for motion as the natural source of relief, and, volition sympathising to the required degree only, the person gets up, and walks till tired: having thus exhausted the muscular and nervous irritation by exercise in the cool night air, he returns to bed, sleeps soundly, and, next day, has no recollection of his nocturnal promenade.

Mesmeric Sleep-walking.—July 18th.—I entranced five men to-day, in the presence of the Rev. Mr. Fisher, and Mr. Clint, Principal of Hooghly college: two of them awoke, on being pulled up, and set on their feet; the others slept standing.

No. 1 could not possibly open his eyes, though he understood my order to do so, and tried with all his might; nor could he walk when desired, but being set in motion, he poked helplessly forward, till he came in contact with the wall, against which he bowed his head, and then stood motionless. Being relieved from his dilemma, and set a-going again, he slouched about, a most forlorn-looking wretch, till he got embayed between a window shutter and the wall, and there he would have remained till the fit went off, if I had not taken pity on him.

No. 2 on being raised, and roused a little by rubbing, and blowing in his eyes, half opened them, and saw sufficiently to enable him to avoid obstacles. Being ordered to walk, he stalked out of the room like a walking corpse; descended four steps, very cautiously, and continued his course in a straight line: when ordered to stop, he did so, and would never have moved again, of his own accord, till the unnatural state disappeared.

No. 3 being roused, opened his eyes wider than natural, but saw no better than the others. I think he even saw less, as he had to be warned of the steps, to prevent his falling: his pupils were dilated, and he never winked. Having got upon the grass, his actions portrayed the most helpless timidity: he walked as if upon glass, and stared intently at every tuft of grass in his way; sometimes turning aside to avoid what, to his disordered senses, probably appeared to be insurmountable obstacles. He turned, when ordered, and made towards the hospital again, picking his steps very cautiously, and never looking up till he came to the steps leading up to the verandah; he then stopped, looked up, carefully studied the nature of the impediment, and, seeing the mass of building before him, gave up the idea of ascending the steps as hopeless, and turned along the road running round the hospital, till he came to where we were standing. Here I stopped him, and very distinctly told him the nature of the obstacle; four steps, namely, and desired him to come to me. This he understood, undertook, and accomplished; being assisted by my warning him at each of the steps, and counting them. All the men, as usual, were unconscious of having left the spot where they went to sleep.

Sleep-waking.—At other times, one or more senses remain active after the others have gone to rest; the wants of the waking organ are transmitted to the sensorium, and are followed by an effort of the will to gratify them. The sleeper rises, and performs the actions necessary to satisfy his desires; eye-sight, to a small extent, usually assists; if not, hearing and touch come to his aid, and guide him with singular accuracy in known localities. I may here give an illustration, from my own experience, of the preternatural acuteness of hearing, developed to aid the somnambulist in getting out of his troubles. In my youth, I was an eager sportsman, by flood and field; and one night, after a fatiguing day's sport, I found myself in the middle of the room, and very cold, but could not possibly contrive to get back to bed again. My last waking impression was made by the ticking of my watch under the pillow, and this recollection came to rescue me from my difficulties. After the most mature reflection, it occurred to me, that if I could only detect my watch by its ticking, I should also find my bed. Acting upon this happy idea, I hunted my watch by ear, till I actually found it; and got into bed again, as the reward of sound reasoning and perseverance.

I may also here notice a similar instance which occurred to my brother, a clergyman in Scotland. I give it in his own words:—"Returning to London, after a tedious and dangerous voyage from the continent, I retired to bed shortly after reaching my hotel. I had taken possession of a spacious apartment, in which were two beds, of which only one was occupied. I soon fell asleep, as I thought, but in a short time left my bed, and wandered about in the greatest perplexity, under the idea that I was still on board the foreign steamer, which I had recently left. I went from berth to berth, as I conceived, beseeching all and sundry to show me my own berth. At last I came in contact with the empty bed, and creeping over it, got embayed between it and the wall. I was long of getting out of this new dilemma, and resuming my supplications to the numerous sleepers by whom I fancied myself surrounded. I remember well one part of the affair, which filled me with the greatest trepidation. I came up to a small table, on which I distinctly heard a watch ticking. The idea came into my head that should the owner awake, and find me in such suspicious proximity to his watch, he would denounce me as a thief. I spoke long and eloquently, rebutting the base suspicion, but the sleeper remained unmoved; I paced about in despair. I came to the door, but having locked it, it did not yield to my attempt at opening; but on coming to the window I drew up the blind, and was still more bewildered on seeing the mighty mass of London spread out before me. The light of the moon, however, striking on the watch, was at last the means of restoring me to the full use of my senses. It suddenly occurred to me that the watch was my own. I instantly seized it, and forthwith was wide awake. I was in the middle of the room, and in a cold sweat. A considerable time must have elapsed, during the occurrences above described, and the curious thing is, that my eyes were wide open the whole time. I spoke only French, and that with the greatest volubility."

Mesmeric Sleep-waking.—The following is a beautiful example of the same condition of mind, produced by art.

Mrs. ———, an English lady, wished to be entranced, to have a tooth taken out by the dentist, who was shortly expected to arrive. I told her husband, that my labour would be in vain, if she thought advantage was going to be taken of her sleep; fear and anxiety being quite destructive to the production of coma; and suggested that when the dentist arrived, I should then propose to make a preliminary experiment, telling her, that if it succeeded she could then suit her convenience, and be entranced at any time, to have the tooth taken out.

The dentist came, and his arrival being carefully concealed from the lady, I proposed to test her powers of submission. At the end of half an hour, her arms appearing cataleptic, I desired her husband to order the carriage, and go for the dentist. In a quarter of an hour they arrived, and I bent back the lady's head, and began to open her mouth without any attempt at resistance; but, on the window being thrown open to give the dentist light, she awoke with a sudden start, and said the dentist was present. She thus described her feelings: she very soon became unconscious, after feeling a general sense of warmth and oppression on the chest; she felt me raise her arms, and leave them in the air without the power to move them, but did not hear me desire her husband to get the carriage ready. She heard the carriage wheels, however, and then it flashed across her brain that her husband had gone to bring the dentist, (although she firmly believed him to be in Calcutta,) and this conviction, from that minute, took complete possession of her mind. She greatly wished to call back her husband, or to get up and run, but she could not move tongue or foot, and showed all the time the most perfect repose of body and feature. She heard the carriage return, and knew it brought the dreaded dentist; was sure it was he who was speaking to her husband, and yet remained fixed to her seat, like a statue. In this instance, the sense of hearing was the only means of communication with the outward world, but it excited a former train of ideas; and how accurately did fear and causality come to a right conclusion, from the ear having transmitted a suspicious sound!

This case opened out to me the nature of Somnambulism, and taught me how to make somnambulists.

Dreaming of the Organs of Sentiment and Intellect.—Perhaps no demand is made on the organs of sense; but the waking parts of the brain are those connected with the passions, feelings, hopes, and fears of the individual. The imagination becomes inflamed by sympathy with the excited organ, and the most vivid sensations of pain or pleasure, ecstacy and agony, are excited, according to the organ stimulated, and the control, more or less, of the reflecting power. The lover, the miser, the philanthropist, and the murderer; the man who hopes for coming good fortune, and he who lives in constant dread of coming evil; all enjoy, or torment, themselves to a height of pleasure, or horror, that cannot be felt when awake. If the reflecting organs are chiefly called into play, then the man of business does a stroke in trade, or conceives a capital speculation that might be of use to him, if he could recollect it when awake: the student easily conquers his difficulties; the mathematician solves the problem, and the historian removes a doubt; the poet's thoughts and lines no longer leave his brain like bird-lime, but he pours forth his soul "in thoughts that breathe, and words that burn." All good dreamers, in fact, confess that they think, say, and do better things when asleep than when awake. Or, let us suppose that the reflecting organs have been intensely engaged during the day, in considering our proper course of action in certain circumstances, and the probable consequences, or that a craving to penetrate the future has been the haunting idea; then the judgment is undisturbed by external impressions, and undistracted by passion, self-interest, and routine habits of thought, and supplied by memory only with the past experience and knowledge that bear upon the question;

under these circumstances it is imaginable that the mind may jump to just conclusions, and receive a clear and happy glimpse into futurity. These impressions, when remembered on waking, and verified by subsequent events, are naturally converted into inspired dreams, and supernatural warnings, merely by the train of reasoning having been lost. The persons, in reality, have reasoned correctly, but by an unusual mode, whose processes have penetrated the future, only by comparing it with the past. In this way

> "Old experience may attain
> To something like prophetic strain."

And such dreams being remembered, and the reasoning analysed, may be of real use to us, in shaping the course of our present and future conduct, because our sleeping conclusions have been come to from just premises, and the natural process of connecting cause and effect: whether this is done sleeping or waking, is of little consequence, the results being equally correct.

If the state of one's health has intensely occupied the thoughts, and the hope of being cured of some distressing complaint is the leading idea; then the man of medical and physical knowledge may possibly hit on the precise nature of his disease in dreaming, and prescribe for its cure in sleep better than he could have done by waking reflection; and, perhaps, the animal instinct of self-preservation may be concentrated on the case, and suggest a course of proceeding, the *rationale* of which we do not understand, but which yet may benefit the patient if acted upon; just as morbid longings, as we call them, (though frequently they are promptings of nature, and ought never to be despised by the physician,) often do the system good, when yielded to and gratified. This is called dreaming of what will do one good.

Mesmeric Dreaming of Different Organs.—As in natural sleep the organs are often preternaturally excited, and their powers singularly increased, by the concentration of the nervous energy upon them; so, in the mesmeric sleep, this may be effected, and of course to a greater and more wonderful extent, by the person being under the control of a reflecting and directing agent, instead of being left to the fitful lights of his own imagination, and the short unsustained flights of his intellect, as in common dreaming. This power of acting on separate portions of the brain, and thereby inducing such trains of thought as we may be pleased to excite, will perhaps be found of practical utility in the treatment of mental diseases; the diseased haunting idea might be banished, and a more healthy tone of feeling and reasoning substituted and sustained, till a new and better habit of mind was produced. I see no reason to doubt that the mental organs can be isolated and exalted by the mesmeric influence under the direction of a skilful leader and suggester, and can readily believe that the mind, by this artificial stimulus, may be excited into more vigorous activity than when acted upon by the usual conditions of life. If persons may derive benefit from night thoughts in dreams, their sleep-waking day thoughts should be more valuable; but the one has no more pretensions to supernatural power than the other. The night-dream is woven out of past impressions lighted up by a flickering imagination and a wavering judgment; and the somnambulist has only the advantage of having his thoughts sustained and concentrated by his mental director. Nor, considering the excessive nervous delicacy developed in the course of mesmeric treatment, and the power of fixing the whole attention upon their bodily sensations, do I think it impossible that somnambulists may acquire an instinctive perception of the condition of their organs, and occasionally be able to prescribe something for their relief; just as persons dream, under nearly an analogous state, of what will do them good, and which sometimes really does so. My psychological experiments have been very limited, partly because I feared to bewilder myself at the outset, and also from want of proper subjects to try them on. The mental range of my patients is so circumscribed, that the topics of food, drink, and clothing, almost exhaust it, and with most of them I have no common language. But I have done enough to show me how the higher grades of somnambulism may be reached; and with more highly organised and intellectual natures, I should have good hopes of doing so.

If properly set about, somnambulism may be produced at a very early stage of the mesmeric phasis, or can be developed as the first step in the return to life from the mesmeric trance; but in the latter case, the sleeper is apt to wake up, at once, to perfect consciousness. To make the simple somnambulist, it is only necessary to operate on the person till his arms become cataleptic; all expression then vanishes, and even when the person answers on subjects of deep interest to himself, no sign of mental emotion ever disturbs his countenance. This statue-like serenity of features may be singularly broken by concentrating his attention, and desiring him to do whatever you do: he then becomes an imitative automaton, mimicking most servilely, and exactly, the actions and words of the mesmerist, or any one substituted for him, and who attracts his attention. Even at this stage, I have not established any "rapport" between the parties, but have only desired the person who took my place to call upon the somnambulist repeatedly by name, till he answered, and then to give clear and short orders, which were obeyed as readily as my own. There is much misapprehension prevalent, I am convinced, about the necessity of "rapport" in the physical and lower mental phenomena of Mesmerism: most of my experiments have been made on patients first entranced by my assistants, and my subsequent control over their movements was often acquired without touching them; it being only necessary for me to attract their exclusive attention.

July 29th.—I made a man senseless and cataleptic, at a great distance, in the presence of a large number of gentlemen, who had come from Calcutta and elsewhere*; among them were six doctors, in whose hands, and in those of the rest of the company, he was left as long as they pleased, without my approaching till I was requested to awake him, after they had all tried in vain. This I did, but only to the extent of enabling him to walk and follow me. I then said, that I would try to clear up his perceptive organs sufficiently to permit him to understand my wishes, with which he would implicitly comply: I did not wish to leave him the power of speech even, at this stage. Having attracted his ear, I ordered him to do what I did, and this he very faithfully performed by throwing himself, on the instant, into every attitude I assumed; but I required to be careful, for if I threw him much out of balance, he was in danger of plunging head foremost against the floor. Those who did not see him, may

*I take the liberty to give the names of such gentlemen as I knew, or who were introduced to me; not, however, as being all vouchers for the truth of Mesmerism, for I did not know many of them, and know not the effect produced on their minds by what they saw. There were upwards of 60 persons present, and some will be found, I hope, to put me right, if I misrepresent, or incorrectly report, what every one saw. Messrs. Barlow, and Tucker, Judges of the Sudder Court; Mr. Elliot, Law Commissioner; Mr. Hardinge, Capt. Hardinge, Mr. Melville, Mr. Larpent, Mr. Bayley, Mr. Wanchope, Mr. Jackson, Mr. Graves, Mr. Clermont, Mr. Betts, the Rev. H. Fisher, the Rev. F. Fisher, the Rev. Mr. Bradbury, Mr. Hunter, Mr. Bennett, Major Wood, Major Anderson, Major Riddell, Capt. Duncan, Capt. Cantley, Dr. McPherson, Dr. Smith, Dr. Burt, Dr. Walker, Dr. Elton, Dr. Ross.

imagine how little the poor fellow knew what he was about, when they were told, that he took the "longitude" of the judges of the Supreme Court with the cool impudence and precision of a cab-man, and the gravity of an astronomer. I then proceeded to free his voice, but only to the extent of making him my echo: he was told to repeat whatever I said, and he showed his intelligence by *repeating the order*. He then gave us "Ye Mariners of England," and if the pronunciation was not very perfect, he seemed to me to reverberate exactly my tones, and my gesticulations were also faithfully copied. We passed suddenly from "grave to gay," and he did such justice to "Hey diddle diddle," that I lost my gravity and burst into a laugh; he joined me in full chorus, and I heard it remarked "he can't help laughing himself;" and some were now quite satisfied that he was found out! upon this, I stopped laughing, and, on the instant, his features relapsed into the most awful repose, and I pointed out that it was no joke to him, but purely imitative laughter, and this, I should think, became evident to all. He also sang "God save the Queen," as well, or rather as badly as I, for he is capable of much better things, under a more skilful music master. I now awoke him up a little more, and made him capable of answering questions: he was asked if he could fence; he said that he could; and I bid him show me. He began to cut the preliminary capers of the native fencers, but, in the act of stooping, a fit of rigidity shot through him, and he would have fallen with dangerous violence against the floor, if his fall had not been fortunately broken. I am always alarmed, and on the look out, when this man is experimented on, from this tendency to instantaneous rigidity of the body. A profound trance, from which it is very difficult to awake him, succeeds such exertions, and usually lasts for four or five hours. I showed another step in the mental phenomena, on other subjects; enabling them to answer simple questions correctly, and extinguishing and releasing the power at pleasure. All reflection being dormant, they feel a natural impulse to give a direct answer to a direct question, and in this way tell me frankly whatever I choose to ask. We are assured that common sleepers can also be played upon in the same way by patient and skilful persons, and that this is well known to the secret police of France.

Catalepsy.—The following is a medical description of natural catalepsy, from the Cyclopædia of Practical Medicine. "The attack is generally instantaneous, the sudden rigidity of the trunk and limbs, the suspension of the senses, and temporary interruption of the exercise of the intellectual faculties, having been preceded by no premonitory stage. The patient retains the posture of body and the expression of countenance which he chanced to have at the moment of seizure; and by this combination of fixed attitude and unvarying expression, presents the air of a statue rather than of an animated being. The eyes continue either fixedly, or shut, as they happened to be at the commencement, whilst the pupil, though usually dilated, contracts on the approach of a strong light. The balance between the flexor and extensor muscles is so perfect, that any new position given to the head, trunk, or extremities, by an external force, is easily received, and steadily maintained. This passive energy of the muscular system, permitting the body to be moulded into almost as great a variety of attitudes as if it were a figure of wax or lead, is the distinguishing characteristic of the disease."

Mesmeric Catalepsy.—Sept. 24th.—Mr. Blyth, curator of the Asiatic Society's Museum, paid me a visit yesterday, and saw various mesmeric operations in my hospitals. He begged so earnestly to be allowed to see a somnambulist that I was over-persuaded to gratify him, as I wished to confine myself to the purely medical relations of Mesmerism. I told him, that when the mesmeric influence, or rather disease, had been deeply felt by the constitution, any body could re-develop it very easily, and that if he would follow my directions, he might mesmerise a man for himself, and convert him into a somnambulist afterwards.

He accordingly rendered a man senseless, standing erect, in a few minutes, and failing to awake him, requested me to do so, which was instantaneously done. But, as often happens, when the system is deeply affected, he fell back into the trance, and Mr. B. begged to see the imitative stage of somnambulism. I said, he could do this also himself, by concentrating the patient's attention. Mr. B. was sitting on a table a few yards in front of the man, and made all kinds of noises, which he echoed back. Wishing to examine him more closely, Mr. B. jumped off the table, and came running forward with his body bent, and singing. The man did exactly the same, but a sudden fit of rigidity passed through him, and he plunged head foremost against the floor, to Mr. B.'s great distress. I had him placed on a comfortable bed to sleep off the effects, and we left him at 1 o'clock, P. M.

I was painfully startled to find the man stiff as a log to-day, at 11 o'clock, and that he had shown no sign of life since we left him.

This would have not alarmed me without the accident, but I feared the head might have been injured by his fall, and set about restoring him to his senses by the usual mesmeric processes, but all in vain. I then had recourse to volatile stimulants to the nose (I could not induce any attempt to swallow,) and effusion of cold water on the body, and to water poured from a height into his open eyes; but to no purpose. I returned in an hour, and renewed my efforts; no fluid could be got to pass down his throat, it ran out of his mouth as from a dead man's; while looking on attentively, I saw an instinctive effort made to clear the wind-pipe of mucus that obstructed it, and then an attempt to swallow; I took advantage of this, and poured some water down his throat; some, luckily for my purpose, passed into his wind-pipe, and brought on a violent fit of spasmodic coughing. I continued to rouse the system at the same time, by every possible means, and succeeded in awaking him. But from the rigidity of the muscles of respiration continuing, his efforts to get rid of the water, and the accumulated mucus of twenty-four hours, nearly choked him. At length, the respiratory muscles resumed their natural action, and enabled him to eject the phlegm from his wind-pipe.

After the trunk had become pliable, his legs remained as rigid as bars of iron, and could not be bent for half an hour afterwards.

This will not only be a lesson to myself, but to others, I hope; and, in future, I must resist all application to do more than is necessary for the removal of disease, even at the expense of being thought uncourteous and disobliging.

Coma.—"Last stage of all in this strange, eventful history," is only separated from the chamber of death by a very fine partition. In this, mind and body are equally torpid, and insensible to all external impressions. It is seen in persons exhausted by long watching and fatigue, exposure to cold, or intense suffering of body and mind; and in this condition of the nervous system surgical operations might often be performed without causing pain. Irregularity in the vital organs, anguish and misery of the countenance, characterise natural coma, and indicate that the icy hand of death is arresting the currents of life, and, in general, the last trump alone can rouse the sleeper from this torpor of exhaustion.

Mesmeric Coma.—In this, the great organic functions are usually undisturbed; the countenance is calm and full, and the complexion that of health. The person is generally easily aroused, and how different is his waking! In an instant, often, he returns to full life and consciousness, without knowing that he has been asleep, and his feelings are often those of pleasure and relief; if he has lain down in pain, he often awakes free from it, and renovated in strength and spirits. In the subsequent part of this work, abundant instances will be given of this, and I will only here introduce one.

May 22d.—I went to-day to see my patient Mr. Clermont, head master of Hooghly College; but found that he had gone out to his duty. Mrs. Clermont mentioned, that she was suffering from one of her nervous headaches, which commence with a pain in the back of the neck, that spreads over the scalp, and around the eye-brows; she had been weakly and nervous of late. She knew nothing about Mesmerism, and I had never mentioned it to her, but now proposed to try the effect of it on her complaint. No objection being made, I requested her to turn her back to me, and sit erect in her chair, and describe anything uncommon she might feel during the process.

After a few minutes, she said that she felt a warmth in the neck, and on extending my manipulations, it advanced to the scalp and eyes. In about eight minutes, she said that the pain was much less, and that she felt very drowsy: upon which, I asked, "shall I put you to sleep?" She only smiled in reply, raised her right arm, put her hand to the side of her head, and went to sleep. At this moment a lady (Mr. Clermont's sister,) entered the room, and I begged her to remain by Mrs. Clermont till I returned with her husband. Having found him, I asked pardon for taking the liberty of mesmerising his wife without his consent, and requested him to return to see her awake. We found her as I had left her, with some members of the family looking on. I extended her arm at a right angle to her body, in which position, or any other, it remained fixed till moved again, and her sister-in-law pricked her hand unheeded. As I saw the party becoming uneasy, I awoke her, but with considerable difficulty: she felt very much ashamed at having been found asleep by me, as she supposed, and it was only after long questioning and reflection that she recalled the circumstances attending her sleep. The headache was quite gone, and she felt, and looked, greatly refreshed.

Letter from Mr. Clermont.

"My Dear Sir,

"I have read your report to the parties who were in the next room at the time you mesmerised Mrs. Clermont. They are perfectly satisfied as to its correctness, and have not the slightest objection to your making use of their names, if necessary. It would be superfluous to detail here the circumstances which came under my observation on my return from Judge Russell's, as they have already been described by you. But, in short, I fully corroborate your account of the case, and even bear the most positive testimony to all that transpired in my presence. You will be glad to learn, that Mrs. Clermont has been doing well ever since. I am, Yours faithfully,

"T. M. Clermont.

"*Chinsurah, May 25th,* 1845.

"P. S. I herein insert the names of the parties present:—

"Miss Clermont.

"Mr. Manly.

"Mr. Philipsz. } Students of the Medical College."
"Mr. Scott. }

Nov. 23.—Mrs. Clermont has not suffered any return of the headache, and no longer feels the distressing languor and oppression she complained of till she was mesmerised.

Natural Clairvoyance.—This is recorded to have been seen in cases of natural catalepsy, and a French physician, M. Petetin, has related several instances of it, which are as well attested as most facts in the history of medicine. M. Petetin had opposed Mesmerism, when alive, and the cases of catalepsy, in which he had observed a transference of the senses, were found among his posthumous papers, and published after his death. In his first case, the discovery was purely accidental: a cataleptic patient was seized with an uncontrollable impulse to sing, which nothing could stop, as she was completely deaf and insensible to external impressions on the organs of sense.

M. Petetin fell by accident across the bed, and when his mouth was near the patient's stomach, exclaimed in despair, "Good God! what a pity that this woman can't be stopped singing!" This exclamation the woman heard, and answered, to his great amazement, and they continued to converse through the pit of her stomach, and the functions of other senses were also performed by remote parts of the body. All this is supported by unexceptionable authority; such as one cannot reject, and hope to be himself believed.

It has also been seen and described by unprofessional persons of intelligence and veracity; of which the following is a curious example: it is a communication from a clergyman to Sir George McKenzie, President of the Edinburgh Phrenological Society, and was written without any reference to Mesmerism, and before it had attracted any attention in England:—

"DEAR SIR,

"It is perfectly true, that our poor friend, who has now been some months with us, presents one of those singular and almost incredible cases of hysterical or nervous affection, which are at distant intervals witnessed under the dispensation of the Almighty. The overthrow of the regular functions of the nervous system was occasioned by the almost sudden death of her father (to whom she was fondly attached,) who was seized with illness, during her absence from him, and died in a few hours after she returned to her home. I cannot enter into any longer details of the case, which has been attended with all those varieties, which have long characterised the complaint among medical men as the Protean disorder. The extraordinary powers communicated to the other senses by the temporary suspension of one or two of them, are beyond credibility to all those who do not witness it: and I really seldom enter into any of the details, because it would be but reasonable, that those who have not seen should doubt the reality of them.

"All colours she can distinguish with the greatest correctness by night or by day, whether presented to her on cloth, silk, muslin, wax, or even glass; and this I may safely say, as easily on any part of the body as with the hands, although, of course, the ordinary routine of such an exhibition of power takes place with the hands,—the other being that of mere curiosity. Her delicacy of mind, and high tone of religious feeling, are such, that she has the greatest objection to make that which she regards in the light of a heavy affliction from God, a matter of show or curiosity to others, although to ourselves, of course, all these unusual extravagances of nervous sensibility are manifest, for at least twelve out of every twenty-four hours. She can not only read with the greatest rapidity any writing that is legible to us, music, &c., with the mere passing of her fingers over it, whether in a dark or light room, (for her sight is for the most part suspended, when under the influence of the attack, or paroxysm, although she is perfectly sensible,—nay, more acute and clever than in her natural state;) but within this month past she has been able to collect the contents of any printing or MS., by merely laying her hand on the page, without tracing the lines or letters; and I saw her, last night only, declare the contents of a note just brought into the room, in this way, (when I could not decipher it myself, without a candle) and with a rapidity with which I could not have read it by daylight. I have seen her develop hand-writing by the application of a note to the back of her hand, neck, or foot; and she can do it at any time. There is nothing unnatural in this, for, of course, the nervous susceptibility extends all over the surface of the body, but use and habit cause us to limit its power more to the fingers. Many, even medical men, take upon themselves to declare, that we are all, her medical attendants as well, under a mere delusion. We ask none to believe anything, if they prefer not to do so, and only reply,—The case is equally marvellous either way; either that this poor patient should be thus afflicted, or that eighteen or nineteen persons of my family and friends, in the daily habit of seeing her, should fancy she is, for every twelve hours out of the twenty-four, doing at intervals that which she is not doing. There are many exhibitions of extravagant powers which she possesses, that we talk of to no one; for finding it difficult to acquire credit for lesser things, we do not venture on the greater. Her power ceases the moment the attack passes off. A considerable swelling has at times been visible at the back of the head, which has yielded to the treatment. It is certainly a case which would be an instructive one, in the consideration of the physiology of the human frame: but she, poor thing! is most averse to experiments being purposely made on her; but in her every day life among us, we have no lack of proof for all we believe and know.

"Between the attacks, she is as perfectly in a natural state as ever she was in her life. There is but one paradox in her state; and that is, that she can, at such times, hear some sounds, and not others, though very much louder, and see some things, and not others, though placed before her. She could hear a tune whistled, when she could not hear a gun fired close to her. It is certainly the absorption or absence of mind that occasions this; absent to some things, though present to others, like any absent man; and thus Dr. Y. accounts for it. In making this communication to you, in part to vindicate the testimony of my friend, Mr. M., I have really exceeded my usual custom and resolution; for

I do not think it fair to the poor sufferer herself, to make her too much the talk of others. Very few believe what we tell them, and therefore we are in no degree anxious to open our lips on the subject. All I know is, that I should not have believed it myself, had I been only told it. I must beg, that you will not make any undue use of this communication, by handing my letter about to any one. The friend for whom you ask the information is perfectly welcome to read it, or I should not have written it. If the case were my own, the world should be welcome to it; but a young female of such sensibility might be much embarrassed by finding the world at large in possession of all particulars on her recovery, should God so please to permit.

"I am, &c. &c.

" ———"

Mesmeric Clairvoyance.—If the above are *facts* (and it is no sign of credulity to believe them till they are refuted, which has never been done, I believe,) I think it extremely probable that art, having copied nature so far, can also imitate her in this; and that clairvoyance has actually been produced in the derangement of the nervous system caused by Mesmerism. It has not yet occurred in my experience, but I should not be at all surprised to encounter it. A gentleman who saw me amputate a tumor, 28 lbs. weight, the other day, and cut and rudely handle the most delicate parts of the human body for twenty minutes without the patient showing a sign of life, said at the conclusion, "Well! I have learned one thing to-day, and that is—never to be again *positive* about anything: I did not believe a word of it, and am now completely convinced of its truth;" and those who wish to know the truth about Mesmerism will do well to follow his example.

It would be more prudent perhaps to continue my facts, and plead ignorance of the *modus operandi* of this mysterious agent; but it is impossible not to think, though perhaps little to the purpose. By turning it all round we may chance to make a happy hit, perhaps; but nothing can be gained by indulging only in thoughtless wonder: I shall, therefore, venture to put down what has occurred to me about it.

The exhaustion of any particular organ, the eye for instance, and the consequent derangement of the nervous system; the shock given to the nervous centres by sudden mental emotions, or the effect produced on the imagination by a powerful mind acting on a weaker; have all been said, and truly, to simulate the mesmeric symptoms, and therefore "imagination" has very generally got the credit of being the "primum mobile" in these singular affections of the system; and I do not intend to dispute its power, or the reality of the effects produced by this agency. But my profound impression is, that the first effects produced on my patients by the mode of practising Mesmerism, are of a purely physical nature; an influence exerted by one animal over another, under certain circumstances and conditions of their respective systems. I should as soon adopt the "opium diabolical," or "all humbug theory," as a satisfactory solution of the problem, as attempt by the action of the imagination to account for what I have seen and done. Would the most imaginative of my readers ever think the following process as a likely means to make people insensible to fire and steel, by the effect produced on the imagination? A Bengal coolie, or pariah, comes before me for the first time, and I see he has a disease requiring a surgical operation; I never say a word to him, but desire my assistants to take him to another room and mermerise him. They desire him to lie down, shut his eyes, and try to sleep, and they pass their hands slowly over the most sensitive parts of the body; exhaling their breath upon the patient, and loading him with their sweat, if he does not readily yield to the mesmeric influence. A few minutes of this will sometimes suffice, but more generally it takes hours, and relays of mesmerisers; and a less imaginative process I cannot imagine. Calomel, rhubarb, and castor oil, have all the same effects, and it seems to me, that it would be as reasonable to say they were *therefore* all the same thing, as to declare the effects of the above process to be "all imagination." "Well! there is *one* thing certain; and that is, that imagination has nothing to do with this," is the common remark of gentlemen who have witnessed the cause and effect, and whose senses are not stuffed by prejudice. That it mingles inexplicably, and inextricably, with the true mesmeric influence, after the constitution has taken on the diseased action deeply, is well known, and will be abundantly shown afterwards; but I now speak of *first effects,* on which alone I desire to insist, in leading proof of the reality and nature of Mesmerism. One person induces mesmeric symptoms by deranging the nervous equilibrium, through a commotion of the mind, another by means of squinting, a third by monotony of sensation, &c.; the same effects being produced by different processes, as we see on many other occasions. It is too common for persons engaged in the same pursuit to become exclusively addicted to their *own way* of gaining their object, and when a new path is open they attempt to obstruct it as an infringement of their exclusive right of way. "Your way is not my way, and therefore it is wrong," argues self-love; and the public seeing so many travellers pretending to reach the same destination, each by his particular route, and every one proclaiming *his* to be the only true road; the impatient public, with its usual slashing logic, sets them all down as wrong, and declares them to be chasing a delusion. Whereas, very often, they are all right, and only wrong by taking too limited a view of the subject: the combined observations of all will probably bring us near the truth, and each plan will be found a useful resource, in different circumstances.

It seems to me that irregularity in the distribution of the nervous energy is at the bottom of all the mesmeric symptoms, however produced, whether naturally or artificially; and I suspect that the same effects may follow a state of exhaustion or repletion of the nervous system. If I might venture on so material an illustration, I should say that the first effects produced in the system by Mesmerism may be likened to a river rolled back upon its source by a heavier body of water, stagnating in its channel, and unable to resume its usual course, till the opposing tide subsides.

From all I have seen, I cannot but believe, that there is an influence of some kind that passes from one person into another, when one of two persons is mesmerised in the way I have described; that, in fact, there is a virtual transfusion of some vital agent from the one body into the other. The wonderful subtlety as well as the effects of this power, lead us to suspect that it is a nervous product; and may it not be the nervous energy passing off by the organs of sense, and even for a short time going beyond the surface of the body; the lungs, meanwhile, and periphery of the body, retaining their vital properties, and remaining under the direction of the will? Every time we move a finger, it is by transmitting *something* under the control of the will to the ends of the fingers, and why should it not go farther? Supposing this to be possible, and that this nervous emanation can be directed by one person upon another, then I would venture to conjecture, that, being a nervous product, it is accepted by the nerves of sense, on coming into contact with them in a continuous well-sustained stream, and is transmitted by them to the brain, thereby adding to, rather than subtracting from, the nervous secretions of the brain, which it is their duty to carry off as soon as formed. If the sensorial secretions are not conveyed away by the nerves of sense and volition, and the exercise of the perceptive and intellectual organs, the brain becomes torpid and oppressed. In like manner, the transmission of foreign nervous matter might overwhelm the brain, or a mere stoppage of its own fluids might steep it in a sleepy drench, and the functions of the sensorium would not be restored until the usual outlet for its energies were re-established.

The entireness of the organic functions would seem to countenance the idea, that the external influence is propagated to the brain by the nerves of sense: the general and capillary circulation, the respiration, and temperature, often remain tranquil, and natural, as in sleep; which shows that organic life is little affected. The accumulation of nervous fluid that oppresses the brain, is also seen in the singular condition of the muscular system, and may perhaps explain the strange helplessness, and at the same time the wonderful passive power of resistance in the muscles, which enables cataleptics to stand asleep in the most painful and exhausting attitudes, longer than would wear out the strongest and most practised athletæ, who enjoy all the resources of art and training. The absorption of another's nervous emanations being thought possible, and this abnormal susceptibility being once established, it is possible to conceive the extreme degree to which this required habit, of transmitting extraneous nervous fluids to the brain, may be developed; and we can comprehend the delicate impressions that would be made by so subtle an agent on such fiue conductors as the nerves of sense; nor, on such a supposition, should it surprise us to be told, that the subject receives at the same time some impressions of the individuality of the agent, and manifests a certain degree of submission to his *will* even. The shades of such an interchange of vitality would be infinite, and probably resemble the effects which we are told can actually be produced by the mere will of the mesmeriser on his patient. I suspect, however, that considerable error exists regarding the power of the *will* in producing the *physical* mesmeric phenomena. People are *willed* to sleep, I believe, by directing our nervous influence upon them, and simply making them the objects of our attention, which is sufficient to impel this influence against them, and, if they have become extremely sensitive to the impression, the usual specific effects will ensue, and they appear to go to sleep in obedience to our will that they should. I have tested this in a variety of ways, by desiring Hindoos, Mussulmans, and Europeans of all professions, merely to concentrate their attention upon certain highly sensitive patients; and the results were as striking and certain as if the most energetic will had been directed against them. On one memorable and ludicrous occasion, I induced a learned brother (who came purposely to expose the "humbug") to give me the command of his person for a short time. The result was, I forced him, *against his will,* and "in spite of his teeth," to produce all the mesmeric symptoms, from the quivering of an eyelid, to the most intense coma, in subjects of morbid sensitiveness, in whom the tendency to mesmeric action had become a deep-rooted disease. The will is no doubt very influential in producing first effects by giving continuity and intensity to our influence, but the system having been once deeply affected, the simple act of attention, on the part of any one, seems to be quite sufficient to bring it within his nervous atmosphere and influence.

But I wish it to be understood, that I speak only of the physical and inferior mental phenomena, such as I have described; of the higher mental manifestations I have no personal knowledge, and to produce them, mental sympathy will no doubt be indispensable. That the nervous sensibility has retreated from the surface, and the organs of sense, is evident to all observers, by the universal insensibility; and the condition of the brain, and muscular system, would seem to indicate that they labour under the effects of this revulsion. The means used to de-mesmerise particular organs, and the brain itself, appear to act by determining the nervous currents back to the surface, thereby relieving the deeper organs from the load that oppressed them; at least I cannot account for the following singular exhibition in any other way.

Nov. 16.—In the presence of Mr. S. Palmer, Major Smith, Mr. Stopford, and Dr. Scott, I showed the spontaneous development of the mesmeric disease (for such it becomes, if pushed far) in a man who becomes entranced to the most intense degree, by being merely brought into my presence: every one was left to test his conditions, in his own way, and no one doubted the *reality* of his condition. I at last awoke him for them, and carrying him to the end of the room, placed him erect against the wall; in a few minutes he relapsed into the trance, and I catalepsed him in the attitude of St. Andrew on the cross. I then mesmerised another man, only, however, to the extent of sealing his eyes, and inducing the cataleptic tendency in the muscles: having set him walking, I extended his arms horizontally, and directed him against the man crucified on the wall. On coming into contact with him, he stopped, and I urged him on, asking "what stopped him?" He tried in vain to separate his eyelids, in order that he might see the nature of the obstruction, and, having no use of his hands, he thought of helping himself by rubbing his forehead against the object before him: this I stopped by pulling back his head, and it remained stiffened in the position I left it. He was now reduced to utter helplessness, as his feet struck nothing but the wall below: I then blew on his neck, thereby immediately releasing it, and on being again urged to tell what was in his way, he began rubbing his forehead against the man, as before. One arm was next freed in the same way; this he brought into play; then the other, and he used both in feeling and rubbing the man all over, with the greatest earnestness, but without a vestige of expression in his countenance. At length, he said there was a man before him. I also showed, that my breath had no specific effect by doing the same thing with a fan; a current of air being all that was required to dissolve the rigidity of the muscles.

Blowing in the eyes is also the most expeditious way of relieving the brain, and restoring its functions; rubbing the eyes, and pouring water from a height are also efficacious, and sometimes are all needed to de-mesmerise the brain. Air, cold, and friction, are natural stimuli to the skin, and the most likely means to restore its sensibility, if diminished; and I imagine that they relax the mucles by determining again to the surface the nervous currents, which had been thrown back upon the muscular system, when I produced its cataleptic condition. I cannot otherwise account for the following singular effects of cold, which, from my patients being naked, I can apply in any way I please. On several occasions, I have entranced persons standing, stript them naked, and catalepsed them in the most painful postures imaginable and in these they would remain an incredible length of time, but let a little cold water be squirted from a distance on any member, and it became instantly relaxed. If both arms were fixed perpendicularly in the air, one after the other was shot down instantly, by a slight stream of water; and if it was directed to the calf of the leg the person fell, as if he had been hamstrung: or if the body was catalepsed, out of the perpendicular, squirting water on the loins would send the patient head foremost against the ground. Blowing on, or rubbing any part had the same effect, but the general torpor is often too deep to exhibit these sensibilities, and such persons are awoke with great difficulty, by the use of all the de-mesmerising agents.

The respiratory nerves of the face are more particularly sensitive to the impressions of air, cold, and friction; indeed the shock given to a somnambulist by blowing in his face simply, often resembles the effects of an actual blow, and is sufficient to awake him; how, I cannot possibly imagine, unless it be by acting as a relief to the brain, by restoring its secretions to their natural channels.

Having followed, and imitated, nature so far, in producing different symptoms according to the extent of the nervous derangement we induce, I see nothing more wonderful in the mesmeric phenomena than in the disturbances that occur in the atmosphere, when the electric relations of the earth and air are changed, and the equilibrium for a time destroyed; but we need not, I suspect, seek for this marvellous agent among the great inorganic powers of nature; for if they are employed, they are so altered and endowed with new vital qualities, by being subjected to the principle of life, that they are no longer recognisable after being converted from their control of brute matter, to be the directing powers of animal life; and I fear the secret lies too near the sources of life and death for man to be permitted to approach it very nearly.

That an agent capable of affecting the physical condition of the brain to such a degree, should have no influence on it as the organ of thought, appears, at first sight, extremely improbable, and we might reasonably expect the production of singular and abnormal mental phenomena, when the influence was directed so as to act principally upon the intellectual organs. Like wine and opium, the extreme degree of the mesmeric influence torpifies the brain, but in smaller quantities, it is a bodily and mental stimulus, and if it be possible to transfuse our cerebral fluid into the brain of another, I see no absurdity in supposing that it may be stamped with our individuality, and may, for a time, induce a synchrony of action between the brains of the giver and the recipient.

But, beyond the simpler manifestations of somnambulism, all is so dark, that to stop short, and wait for farther evidence, is better than to advance and step in the dark. The ignorance and presumption of man; his passion for the mysterious and marvellous, his powers of self-delusion, with the pranks of knaves and the simplicity of fools, have so mystified the subject, that the artificial difficulties cost us more trouble to remove than the natural; and a mass of rubbish must be removed before we can reach the foundation stone of truth.

CHAPTER V.

The Mesmeric Processes.—Publicity the best Security to the Public.—Ignorance and Indifference the real Dangers.—Mesmeric Treatment of Disease a Field for the Philanthropist.—Puysegur and Deleuze, unprofessional Men.—Processes for producing Coma.—Tumour in Upper Jaw removed during Coma.—Hypertrophy of Scrotum, ditto.—Trance renewable at Pleasure.—Three consecutive Operations on one Person.—Mode of Mesmerising in Chronic Diseases.—Cure of Rheumatism and Nervousness.—Local Mesmerising.—Mesmerised Water.—Process for preparing it.—First experiments with it.—The last.—Means of awaking Persons Mesmerised.

At the commencement of my mesmeric experiments, I had resolved to communicate only to professional men the modes which I had found most effectual in educing the influences of Mesmerism. I was, at first, alarmed at the possible dangers to the public, were the most effectual means of producing the extreme degrees of Mesmerism generally known; but I am now of opinion that the greatest danger to a community is a contemptuous disregard of an unseen and unknown enemy, and, therefore, all I know on this important subject shall be revealed. The best means of avoiding danger is to know its full extent, and, sometimes, the best policy is to meet it half way, fully prepared to repel it. While the public remain in a listless indifferent humour about Mesmerism, the dangers from an abuse of it are very likely,—I may say are very certain—to occur. But when, by attending to the following directions, proofs of its truth shall pour in from every quarter, then Mesmerism will come home to men's minds as a reality, and become an object of personal interest to all; and the instinct of self-preservation will rouse people to take the necessary steps for deriving all the benefit, and avoiding all the danger attending its practice. If evil arises, let the blame rest on the culpable negligence of the public, and the punishment fall on those who pervert good to evil.

The utmost publicity is most consonant to my taste, and, upon the whole, the best security to the public.

Many benevolent and honourable unprofessional persons may

also be induced to exercise their natural gifts, in the alleviation of human suffering, under the superintendence of the physician, who cannot spare the time, and waste of body, which are required before his patients can be benefitted by the processes of Mesmerism. The persons to whom Europe owes its knowledge of Mesmerism, uncontaminated by self-interest and the devices of quackery, were unprofessional men, the Baron Puysegur and M. Deleuze; the one a wealthy French nobleman, who consecrated his life to relieving the sufferings of the poor, and who said it was his mission to lodge Mesmerism in the hands of the doctors (a trust they have been very neglectful of, unfortunately;) and the other, a truthful and benevolent man of letters, long keeper of the "*Jardin des Plantes,*" at Paris, who practised the art for thirty-five years, and whose works are most honest and true guides; errors of judgment, to which all are subject, being their only defects; as I have tested by experience, before reading them.

Coma—I usually procure in the following manner, and am inclined to think that its comparative rarity in Europe is owing to the mesmeric influence not being at once sufficiently concentrated on the patient, by transmitting it to his brain from all the organs of the operator, and through every channel by which it can be communicated. With the necessary degree of patience, and sustained attention, the following process is so effectual in producing coma, that in a large enough field, and with properly instructed assistants, it may here be obtained daily, for the purpose of procuring insensibility to surgical operations. No trial under an hour should be reckoned a fair one; two hours are better; and the most perfect success will often follow frequent failures, but insensibility is sometimes induced in a few minutes.

Desire the patient to lie down, and compose himself to sleep, taking care, if you wish to operate, that he does not know your intention: this object may be gained by saying it is only a trial; for fear and expectation are destructive to the physical impression required. Bring the crown of the patient's head to the end of the bed, and seat yourself so as to be able to bring your face into contact with his, and extend your hands to the pit of the stomach, when it is wished; make the room dark, enjoin quiet, and then shutting your patient's eyes, begin to pass both your hands, in the shape of claws, slowly, within an inch of the surface, from the back of the head to the pit of the stomach; dwelling for several minutes over the eyes, nose, and mouth, and then passing down each side of the neck, go downwards to the pit of the stomach, keeping your hands suspended there for some time. Repeat this process steadily for a quarter of an hour, breathing gently on the head and eyes all the time. The longitudinal passes may then be advantageously terminated, by placing both hands gently, but firmly, on the pit of the stomach and sides;—the perspiration and saliva seem also to aid the effect on the system.

It is better not to test the patient's condition by speaking to him, but by gently trying if the cataleptic tendency exists in the arms. If the arms remain fixed in any position they are left in, and require some force to move them out of every new position, the process has been successful; the patient may soon after be called upon by name, and pricked, and if he does not awake, the operation may be proceeded with. It is impossible to say to what precise extent the insensibility will befriend us: the trance is sometimes completely broken by the knife, but it can occasionally be reproduced by continuing the process, and then the sleeper remembers nothing; he has only been disturbed by a night-mare, of which on waking he retains no recollection. Here is an instance of this.

July 29th.—In the presence of some sixty gentlemen, who came from Calcutta and the vicinity, I to-day cut off an enlarged and ulcerated prepuce; the man moved, and cried out, before I had finished, but was immediately thrown back into the trance, from which all the efforts of the spectators, six doctors included, could not arouse him, or excite a sign of vitality. He was operated on, at twelve o'clock, and awoke at three: on being questioned, he said, that he had felt no pain, and had not seen an European that day. Next day, he complained of the pricks of pins, inflicted upon him by my visitors, who had actually made a pincushion of him. In future, I must request that pins be left at the door.

The person can be raised into any position required for the operation; but some peculiarity in the case may demand the sitting posture from the commencement, as in the following instance.

June 3d.—Teencowrie Paulit, a peasant, aged 40. Two years ago, he began to suffer from a tumour in the antrum maxillare; the tumour has pushed upon the orbit of the eye, filled up the nose, passed into the throat, and caused an enlargement of the glands of the neck.

I was very desirous to reduce him to a state of insensibility before operating on him, and for the last fortnight my assistants have all perseveringly tried it, but without inducing sleep even. Indeed, from the tumour obstructing his throat, he has hardly slept for five months. Having ascertained that he was easier when sitting, I took him in hand myself, to-day, and entranced him in a chair by the following process. The room being darkened, I suspended my spread hands over his head for some time, and then carried them slowly down, one in front, the other behind; the former dwelling over the eyes, nose, mouth, and sides of the neck, and the latter being applied over the base of the brain: both were then carried down the centre of the body, claw-like, to the pit of the stomach, where they were spread and gently pressed, one opposite the other; and I kept breathing on the head and eyes all the time. In half an hour, the man was catalepsed, and in a quarter more, I performed one of the most severe and protracted operations in surgery; the man was totally unconscious.

I put a long knife in at the corner of his mouth, and brought the point out over the cheek-bone, dividing the parts between; from this, I pushed it through the skin at the inner corner of the eye, and dissected the cheek back to the nose. The pressure of the tumour had caused the absorption of the anterior wall of the antrum, and on pressing my fingers between it and the bones, it burst, and a shocking gush of blood, and brain-like matter, followed. The tumour extended as far as my finger could reach under the orbit and cheek-bone, and passed into the gullet—having destroyed the bones and partition of the nose. No one touched the man, and I turned his head into any position I desired, without resistance, and there it remained till I wished to move it again: when the blood accumulated, I bent his head forward, and it ran from his mouth as if from a leaden spout. The man never moved, nor showed any signs of life, except an occasional indistinct moan; but when I threw back his head, and passed my fingers into his throat to detach the mass in that direction, the stream of blood was directed into his wind-pipe, and some instinctive effort became necessary for existence; he therefore coughed, and leaned forward, to get rid of the blood; and I supposed that he then awoke. The operation was by this time finished, and he was laid on the floor to have his face sewed up, and while this was doing, he for the first time opened his eyes.

June 4th.—This is even a more wonderful affair than I supposed yesterday. The man declares by the most emphatic pantomime, that he felt no pain while in the chair, and that when he awoke, I was engaged in sewing up his face, on the floor;—so that the coughing and forward movement to get rid of the blood, were involuntary, instinctive efforts, to prevent suffocation.

June 6th.—The dressings were undone to-day, and the whole extent of the wounds in the face has united completely by the first intention. He is out of all danger, and can speak plainly: he declares most positively, that he knew nothing that had been done to him until he awoke on the floor, and found me sewing up his cheek;—and I presume he knows best. Here is a translation of his own statement in Bengalee:—

"For two years I laboured under this disease, and scarcely slept for five months. On the 19th May, I came to the Imambarah Hospital, and three or four persons tried to make me sleep, but all in vain. On the 3d June Dr. Esdaile having kindly undertaken my cure, with a great deal of labour, made me sleep, and took something out of my left cheek, which at that time I did not perceive. After the operation, I did not sleep for two nights, but after the third day, I have slept as usual.

"TEENCOWRIE PAULIT,
of Madra."

If patients are fortunate enough to sleep some time after the operation, they not only feel no pain on waking, but none subsequently even. The following is an extraordinary instance of the absence of pain, from first to last.

Sept. 1st.—Teg Ali Khan, a tall strong-looking man; has a hypertrophied scrotum, caused by repeated operations for hydrocele by native doctors; who only withdraw the water as often as it accumulates, without attempting the radical cure. The tumour is perfectly round, and as big as a man's head. He was mesmerised in two hours, on the first trial, and, in the presence of Drs. Ross and Sissmore, I dissected out all the parts; which was very tedious, from the testes having contracted adhesions all round them; and it was about half an hour before the organs were covered up again by stitching flaps over them. Not a quiver of the flesh was visible all this time, and at the end, his body was as stiff as a log, from head to foot, and his separated legs could be with difficulty put together again. He awoke in half an hour after the operation, and felt no pain.

Sept. 4th.—The stitches were taken out to-day; the wound has healed throughout, and he has had *no pain whatever* since the operation;—so much for the absence of the usual irritative shock to the system.

We can renew the trance at pleasure, in order to render people insensible to repeated operations.

Sept. 18th.—Morally Dass, a peasant, aged fifty, has an unhealthy cartilaginous sore, half an inch high above the skin, and extending for six inches along the outer ham-string of the left leg, which it has contracted to nearly a right angle with the thigh, for a year past.

He was entranced to-day, for the first time, and I deeply cauterised the whole sore with a red-hot plaister iron, without awaking him.

Sept. 19th.—The excrescence is so hard, and thick, that it must be dissected off the ham-string: he was again entranced, and the diseased part was pared down to a level with the surrounding skin, without his feeling it.

Sept. 20th.—When he was in the trance to-day I straightened the leg completely, and bound it up in splints: he awoke not, and when he did, had no pain; although it took all my strength and weight to break down the adhesions, which I felt and heard cracking under my hands. The Rev. Mr. Bradbury saw the first operation. The Rev. Mr. Fisher, and Mr. Graves, the second, and Mr. Blyth the third. In the treatment of chronic diseases suited for Mesmerism, *coma* is not required: if it occurs, it is probably because nature needs it; but we ought to be satisfied with the improvement of the patient, though it is unaccompanied with any striking phenomena. The system is not less effectually recruited, because it is done silently,—just as the best digestion is least felt. For refreshing the nervous system, and inducing natural sleep, mesmerising "*a longs courants,*" as the French call it, it will be found sufficient. These are steady continuous tractions, with the point of the spread fingers, from head to foot; the head may be occasionally breathed upon, and the hands allowed to rest for a few minutes on the pit of the stomach. An hour of this, on going to bed, will often soothe restlessness, bring back natural sleep, and invigorate the nervous system.

Sept. 25th.—Mr. Calder (I mention his name at his own request,) who has been twenty years in India, came to me to-day, complaining of general rheumatism, nervousness, and debility. He walks with great difficulty, with the help of a stick, and cannot ascend a stair. His nerves are shattered, his eye-sight is weak, and his hands tremble when writing; when he walks on smooth ground, he fancies that it slips from below him, and the effort made to save himself nearly throws him down: of late he has not been able to drive his buggy, from a feeling that it is impossible for him to prevent his horse from running into any carriage he meets. He has been in this state for two years and a half; during which he has gone a tour of doctors, and swallowed a dispensary of physic, to no good purpose. I said that I could not in conscience physic him more, but recommended him to try what nature would do for him, as, upon the whole, I thought his case adapted for mesmeric treatment, but that it would require time and patience to do him any good. He was very glad of any untried chance of relief, and I desired one of my people to mesmerise him for an hour in bed, every night.

Never having been present when Mr. Calder was mesmerised, I am indebted to him for the following note of his case.

"On the 25th of September last, your native assistant, as directed by you, made the first attempt to induce the mesmeric sleep, but without success: the trial lasted for an hour and a half.

"26th and 27th September, ditto.

"28th.—After a persevering trial for the same length of time, I was thrown into a trance, from which I awoke after upwards of five hours,—I found great difficulty in raising my eyelids, or keeping my eyes open. I left the couch and retired to bed, and had my natural sleep afterwards, till six o'clock next morning. For a week afterwards, the efforts to mesmerise me were repeated for an hour daily, but without farther effect than causing a sleep of a few minutes. I however continued to enjoy my natural rest at night, found my pains abating daily, and my nerves considerably braced up; so much so, that I could walk up and down stairs without assistance, and with every confidence drive out in a buggy alone, which I could not have attempted for two years and a half previously.

"Up to the 17th of Oct. I was thrown into sleep, every third or fourth night, for about two hours; the effect of which you may judge of, from my being able to walk yesterday morning more than four, and this morning, more than six miles.

"(Signed) J. CALDER.

"Oct. 28th, 1845."

This is the gentleman who, I said, recognised the identity of the mesmeric processes with the Indian modes of charming away pain.

Topical mesmerising,—by suspending the ends of the fingers over the pained part, breathing on it at the same time, and then drawing the fingers downwards, continued for a long enough time, say an hour or two,—is often very effectual in soothing local pain; and I have seen it relieve the pain in gout, bruises, and rheumatism.

The much ridiculed "mesmerised water" is another means of producing the mesmeric symptoms, and as it is practically useful, the process for preparing it shall be described; and let those who do not choose to avail themselves of it, let it alone. But before doing this, and illustrating its effects by facts, it will perhaps be advisable to clear the way for the reception of them, by showing that there is no *prima facie* absurdity or impossibility about the matter. In accordance with Lord Bacon's advice, I will "foment the part to make the unguent enter the better." To those who will condescend to think seriously on the subject, and apply their previous knowledge to the examination of it, I would suggest, that if there is a vital emanation from the body, called "Mesmerism," there is nothing improbable in the assertion that it can be communicated to water and other inorganic substances, like other invisible and imponderable agents. Water absorbs air and different gases, and the odours of neighbouring objects with great facility; a glass of water can be charged with electricity, or an empty glass filled with it. Mesmerism has been called "animal electricity," and if correctly named, we should expect it to resemble inorganic electricity in many particulars: but whether it is a modification of electricity or not, I can see no reason why water should not absorb an invisible animal fluid, as easily as a fluid which is imperceptible and organic. There is nothing in the known laws of physics to make it improbable that water can be mesmerised, as well as electrified. On the contrary, it seemed to me so probable from analogy, that I fully believed the statements of others regarding it, and made my first experiments with considerable confidence.

Deleuze, a most honest and trustworthy man, and who had practised Mesmerism, for thirty-five years in France, with great success, gives the following directions for mesmerising water. "It is to be poured over the tips of the fingers, and the glass is then to be mesmerised by passing the hands down its sides, and the water may also be breathed upon." The following process, though less delicate, is a shorter, and, I believe, a more effectual mode of charging water with the mesmeric fluid.

As there is good reason to believe that the breath is impregnated with the vital fluid, I breathe through a tube into the bottom of a cupful of water, keeping the points of the fingers in contact with the surface; in five minutes the water is charged, and here are my first experiments with it.

June 28th.—From her extreme sensibility to the influence, it seemed to be probable that the woman Alunga would exhibit in perfection the virtues of mesmerised water, if it had any. In the presence of my hospital attendants, I to-day took an ounce of water from the common reservoir, and mesmerised it, putting the like quantity of plain water into another glass. We then went into the women's ward, and I gave the plain water first very slowly, asking her if it had any taste? It was only plain water, she said; I then gave her the other; after waiting some time, she said it was different from the first,—that it was sharp to the tongue, and created a warmth in the stomach. Almost immediately, her countenance began to change; she insisted upon getting up to walk; and I immediately saw that she was a somnambulist: after taking a few staggering steps, she would have fallen, but was prevented, and taken back to bed, where she instantly sank into the mesmeric coma, and remained so for hours.

June 29th.—I to-day had the pleasure of meeting the Rev. Mr. Long, from Calcutta, a stranger to me and mesmerism, who asked me if I could show him any mesmeric cases in the hospital at present. I replied that I should be happy to verify, in his presence, an important experiment regarding the efficacy of mesmerised water, which I had made for the first time, yesterday. I was glad to learn that he had never heard of such a thing; and he willingly agreed to accompany me to the hospital.

I took the same quantity of water as yesterday, out of the common cistern, and charged it before him, and again put the same measure of plain water in another glass, the woman being unconscious of our presence. We then went to her, administered the common water first, and waited for the effects; none appearing, the mesmerised water was given, and in a few minutes her expression altered; she rose, and walked in a wavering uncertain manner, and then set about washing the floor, which was dirty, she said. Soon after she complained of the room being full of kites, crows, and paddy birds, and desired them to be scared away. On being asked who I was, she said I was a Baboo, and that the sweeper was her brother Essan, who had come to take her home;

she was put to bed, and immediately fell into the mesmeric trance. We then retired to talk over the matter, and I asked Mr. Long if he had any doubts that could be resolved on the spot. He said, nothing could be more certain than the connection of cause and effect, and that he would gladly certify to it. After some time we returned to her, and I awoke her, all but her eyes; these she could not open; but this being done with my assistance, she was seen to be in complete possession of all her senses and faculties, as was evinced by her ready and consistent replies, and the total revolution in her countenance.

June 30th.—I thought of varying the experiment on the woman Alunga, whom I had not seen to-day: I therefore went to the house of my assistant, and asked him to give me a phial and a little water, telling him my intentions, which were to call for Mr. Betts, the deputy-collector (who had never seen Mesmerism and to whom I had never spoken on the subject,) and request him to go to the hospital, give the water to the woman, and then send to inform me that it was done. Having mesmerised the water, I carried the phial to Mr. Betts, and begged him to be good enough to perform an experiment for me, and at the same time satisfy his curiosity, perhaps. I assured him, on my honour, that this was pure water, only mesmerised, and requested him to go and give it to the woman named Alunga, and then to let me know. He kindly consented, and in a short time a messenger came for me; when I arrived, the woman was getting up to walk, in the same delirious state as on former occasions, her phantasms only being varied; and again she could not open her eyes, even by pulling: when partially opened they instantly closed again, till I relieved her by blowing and rubbing. On awaking there was no vestige of derangement in her mind or perceptions. Mr. Betts was sure of the facts he had witnessed, but, I suspect, had some difficulty in believing that *he had only given water*.

June 28th.—Sidissur Ghose, a prisoner, in a different hospital; I saw him for the first time to-day, at 11 o'clock; he has been suffering for three days from inflammation of the testes, which were extremely tender to the touch, and he was bent double in walking. I determined to subject him to the trance if possible, for the following reasons. As a fire expires for want of fuel, it seemed to me very probable that inflammation would die out during many hours of absolute repose to the system, pain and irritation being the sustaining causes of inflammation. Remove all pain and sensibility for hours, and it is only natural to suppose that the circulation will return to its usual channels, and the disease be removed by a natural curative effort. If the repose be too short to recruit the vital powers, the trance can be repeated at will when the system has been once affected. I succeeded in entrancing him in half an hour, and left him sleeping. I then went to the Charity Hospital, and made my first experiment, as above related, on the woman Alunga, with mesmerised water. Having completely succeeded, I returned to the Jail Hospital, and found that the man Sidissur had just awoke. He bore pressure much better, and there was no heat in the part. I gave him three ounces of mesmerised water, and in five minutes he was again in the trance.

June 29th.—Sidissur awoke at nine o'clock last night, but went to sleep again immediately, and slept all night; the swelling has decreased, and I can squeeze the part all over without causing pain, and he walks erect, with ease. The disease is subdued, but for the sake of experiment I gave him another dose of mesmerised water, and in three minutes he was in the trance.

June 30th.—Sidissur again slept till nine o'clock last night, and had a good night afterwards. Dismissed cured, at his own request.

July 2d.—Nobee, an elderly, worn-out woman, has had rheumatism in her back for some months: she was put into the trance to-day, and on waking was free of pain.

July 3rd.—No pain. Gave her a dose of mesmerised water; she soon said that she felt warm all over; a general tremor followed; and on being desired to walk she complained of her head turning, and walked a little, with great difficulty. On returning to bed she fell asleep immediately, and slept for two hours.

July 29th.—At the public Seance, already mentioned, eight men drank mesmerised water prepared by my assistants, and superintended by two doctors, and two clergymen; and in spite of the incessant tormenting of their visitors, four of them, to my great surprise, became entranced and cataleptic, and were converted into somnambulists.

December 14th.—Jadoo, a prisoner, convalescent from cholera, is plagued with continual hiccough—eight convulsions in a minute. To be mesmerised: he was subdued in fifteen minutes, but there was little change in the hiccough for half an hour afterwards. He was raised upon his feet, and a bandage soaked in cold water wound around his chest, without awaking him, and he was allowed to sleep half an hour longer: still no change for the better. I now prepared some mesmerised water, and awoke him; he no sooner drank it than he fell asleep again, and the hiccough immediately stopped, and never returned. He slept for three hours after drinking the water.

To illustrate the subject farther, as I could do by scores of examples, would be intolerably tedious; and I hope it will not be for a moment supposed that I mean to say that such will in general be the effects of mesmerised water, but only that in persons *already under* the mesmeric influence such results can be procured: it has been known to affect the uncontaminated system, but it is a rare occurrence.

The means used for dissipating the mesmeric influence, are precisely those employed for disengaging the brain in fainting, or natural insensibility, caused by a revulsion or stoppage of the nervous fluid by natural causes. They act, I presume, exactly in the same way, by re-determining the nervous rousing to the skin and the organs of sense; thereby rousing the brain from its torpor of exhaustion in the case of fainting, or relieving it of the nervous plethora which I have suggested might be the cause of mesmeric coma.

Blowing sharply in the eyes, rubbing the eye-lids, and eye-brows, and sprinkling cold water in the face, are the methods for de-mesmerising the brain, and when locally applied, are equally efficacious in de-catalepsing rigid limbs. Let an arm be catalepsed, short of the most intense degree of coma, and although it may require considerable force to bend it, yet blowing on it, rubbing it gently, or letting a few drops of cold water fall on it, will generally relax the rigidity of the muscles, and cause the arm to fall down at the side, with its flexibility restored; and it looks to me as if the muscles recovered their functions (just as the activity of the brain is renewed) by being relieved of the nervous secretions that have deserted the surface, and become concentrated on the sensorium and muscular system.

The smallness of the cause, and the greatness of the result, when we restore a person to the complete possession of his senses, and intellect, by sprinkling water in his eyes when in the mesmeric coma, are quite as remarkable in natural fainting, in which the effects are often equally striking and instantaneous; and I leave it to the reader to determine whether the exhaustion of the nervous system in natural coma, and its presumed repletion in the mesmeric state, does not assist us in understanding the similarities and differences observed in natural, and mesmeric sleep.

CHAPTER VI.

Mesmerism as a Remedy.—Coma as a Medical Agent.—Journal of Practical Mesmerism.—Chronic Inflammation of Eye cured.—Nervous Headache ditto.—Acute Inflammation of Eye ditto.—Return of Nervous Headache prevented.—Rev. Mr. Fisher's Report.—How to make a Convert.—Tooth drawn in the Trance.—Convulsions cured by ditto.—Arms straightened in ditto.—Sense of Formication removed.—Lumbago, Sciatica, Pain in Crural Nerve, cured.—Palsy of an Arm ditto.—Hemiplegia greatly benefitted.—Tic cured.—Rheumatism ditto.—Mesmerism as a Disease.—Resembles Hysteria.—Ignorant Charges of Imposture.—The Public abused.—The Public disabused.—Folly and Unfairness of its would-be Guides.—Spontaneous Development of the Mesmeric Disease.—Mesmerising by doing nothing taught by the Mesmerists themselves.—A natural Consequence of frequent Mesmerising.—Examples of Mesmerising by doing nothing.—Hysteric Theory.—Hope to hear of Hysteria as a Remedy soon.—Rational Mode of studying Mesmerism.

For practical purposes, the physical effects of Mesmerism may be divided into simple somnolence, semi-insensibility, and total insensibility, or coma: of the first, nothing more need be said, and abundant examples of the others will be given in my "Journal of Practical Mesmerism."

Although accepting thankfully whatever nature deigned to offer in answer to my inquiries, in the various cases in which I consulted her; yet they were not presented to the *vis medicatrix naturæ,* at haphazard, and without selection. My first case was indeed a "pomegranate full of many kernels," and offered so many facts from which great practical deductions could be drawn, that I only followed out the indications of nature in all my subsequent proceedings; so that my operations have not been "A mighty maze, and all without a plan."

I. I was certain (if life is not a phantasmagoria) that in the mesmeric trance, the muscles of the whole body had been as plastic, and obedient to my command, as clay in the hands of the potter; and I felt satisfied that if the same state of things could be brought about, muscular spasms and contractions would disappear before this great solvent. The straightening of limbs, long contracted, very soon verified this inference.

II. Having, in this case, witnessed the total extinction of nervous irritability, I was led to conclude, that in a like state of things, nervous pains would vanish before this supreme anodyne. The cure of nervous headaches immediately demonstrated the truth of this idea.

III. The insensibility to pain convinced me that the most painful surgical operations might be performed without the knowledge of the patient, and this has been done to an extraordinary extent, so much so, as to be a daily matter of course.

IV. I had seen high local inflammation, and sympathetic fever suspended during the trance in my first patient, and that the artificial inflammation (which it was my object to excite, for the cure of hydrocele,) did not develop itself, while the mesmeric influence was in activity, and that the pulse and temperature had become natural: thence I inferred, that inflammation was probably incompatible with such a state of the constitution, and I soon succeeded in curing acute inflammation of the eye and testis, by no other means than the mesmeric trance.

As regards the certainty of my conclusions, it required no great sagacity to believe the evidence of my senses, and to go and do as nature bid me. A *fact* in nature being once ascertained, and all its accessories carefully observed, we may be confident of re-producing it, at will, by fulfilling the necessary conditions, if the phenomenon is under human control. I therefore tried to bring about the same condition of body, by the means required to be used by nature, before she will condescend to interfere in our favour, feeling convinced that if she did interfere, it would be with unerring wisdom, and unapproachable skill; and that what had been feebly begun by her weak, but obedient creature, would be triumphantly completed by her laws, when brought into action; the way for them being merely prepared, in the manner pointed out by experience.

"Nature is but a name for an effect, whose cause is God;" and the Author of nature has ordained, that such effects should often follow such predisposing causes.

Mesmeric coma will in the following pages chiefly figure in surgical operations, and is not so often required in the treatment of medical cases; but when it can be induced, it is extremely important in instantly extinguishing nervous pains, arresting convulsions, and aiding the natural resolution of inflammation, by its anodyne and restorative powers; and if it could be induced in the commencement of some of the most fatal diseases, it would probably arrest their progress, for it revolutionises the whole system, and every other constitutional affection is for the time suspended.

In chronic inflammation it is a useful discutient, gently stimulating the nerves, and capillary vessels of the part, to more healthy action; and for this purpose, local Mesmerism is only required.

The chronic exhibition of Mesmerism as a general tonic, in diseases of debility promises to be of great service, especially in functional derangement of the nervous system and I am hopeful that we have at last got a *direct* nervous remedy, hitherto, a "desideratum" in medicine.

In palsy from weakness of the nerves, it promises to assist us greatly, and Dr. Elliotson has recorded many cures of cases he could not have managed before. All who venture to confess the truth to themselves, know how miserably impotent for the cure of palsy, and nervous diseases generally, are the medical means hitherto employed. If we succeed, we often cannot tell why, and the connection of cause and effect is very uncertain. But in the chronic treatment of palsy, by Mesmerism alone, the patient often feels and shows early and continued improvement under the action of this natural remedy; and we cannot refuse to believe that it is the exciting cause: we must believe that it is, or own that it is a spontaneous cure of a commonly incurable disease! But both the practitioner and the patient must remember; that Mesmerism is no exception to the general rule, that a chronic disease must have a chronic cure: much patience and labour will be required in the mesmeric treatment of paralytic affections, and the result will greatly depend upon whether the disease is one of debility or over-excitement of the nervous system. In the latter case, I should think, that unless the sedative effects on the system could be induced, we should be disappointed; in the former, every degree of the influence would probably be of service.

We find in practice, that nervous persons, from over-excitement of the nerves, are with great difficulty subdued, and appear to be still farther irritated by subjecting them to the mesmeric process; whereas those who suffer from irritability of the nerves from weakness, are easily affected, and soon benefitted by it.

The medical cases adapted for the use of Mesmerism, do not occur in my practice among the poor so often as surgical cases, as the labouring poor do not usually resort to medical advice for nervous diseases, till they are past cure: I can however present the reader with some interesting cases, which I will extract, as they occurred from my

JOURNAL OF PRACTICAL MESMERISM.

"May 7th.—Nazir, a Mussulman; aged 20: is suffering from the *sequelæ* of ophthalmia of two months' standing; the sight of the left eye is destroyed. The cornea of the right eye is muddy with superficial ulcerations, and a pterygium is forming; there is constant lacrymation, and he cannot distinguish a white man from a black. I placed him in a chair before me, and directed the operation to the eyes and head generally, desiring him to mention what he felt as we proceeded. He soon said, that he felt an agreeable warmth where my fingers passed without touching him; shortly after, he said his eyes were easier, and on extending the process to the body, he felt a general warmth pervade it, and sweat stood in drops on his face. He next said, that he felt a fear come over him that he could not account for, and desired greatly to sleep: having no desire to go farther, I here stopped:—the eyes to be mesmerised daily for ten minutes, and then be put to sleep."

"May 22d.—Has been mesmerised daily, and put to sleep twice: he always feels better after the process; says that his body feels pleasant and light, and the expression of his countenance is much improved. The lacrymation has ceased, and he read two words in Bengalee and Persian to-day; the pterygium will be the only impediment to his sight.

"May 22d.—Keenoo, a prisoner; saw him for the first time to-day, at 11 o'clock. He has had a severe pain extending from the left eye-brow to one half of his head for four days; and there is pain on pressing at the supra-orbitor notch. I made him lie down, in a small room off the hospital, and in twenty minutes left him asleep with one arm raised perpendicularly in the air, and locking the door, I left him alone.

"I returned at 1 o'clock, and on opening the door, found him lying exactly as I had left him with his arm still in the air: he awoke whilst I was looking at him, and said that he had not been asleep. On being asked why his arm was in the air, he could give no reason for it. So sensible is the approach of sleep under this grand narcotic, or so sudden its invasion, that in the minds of the sleepers often no trace remains of the circumstances attending their sleep! This was seen in the case of Mrs. Clermont. He awoke perfectly free from headache.

"May 24th.—No return of pain—discharged cured.

"May 24th.—Nazir Mahomed, a prisoner; saw him for the first time to-day, at 11 o'clock. For the last four days, he has laboured under acute inflammation of the conjunctiva: the conjunctival vessels form a raised zone around the cornea; there is a constant lacrymation, pain over half the head, and he cannot distinguish objects.

"I made him lie down on the floor, and rendered him cataleptic in twenty minutes; then putting his hands, clasped, above his head, I locked the door, and took the key with me to Chinsurah, two miles off, where I found the Rev. Mr. Fisher, and Mr. Money, the collector, who are much interested in my proceedings, and daily ask, 'What progress?' I answered, that a man entranced was waiting my return; and they offered to go back with me. On opening the door we found the man had just awoke; and being asked in what attitude he found himself on waking, he said that his hands were clasped over his head: he reports the pain to have quite left the side of his head; only a little remains about the eye; the eyelids move much more freely, and the watering is less; his general feelings are much improved: before the sleep he felt his body hot and heavy, and it is now cool and light. Cold water to the head and eyes; a dose of physic. When we were leaving the hospital the native doctor reported that a man had just come in with a pain in one side of his head, like the man cured on the 23rd. I desired him to be brought before us, and he stated that for the last six days he had suffered from an acute intermittent headache, confined to one side of his head; that it commences at 4 o'clock in the morning, and continues till 12 P. M. Turning to my friends, I observed that if they would wait I should like to entrance this man, as a preventive. They consented to do so, and Mr. Fisher has been good enough to send me his notes of what followed:—

"Mr. Fisher's Report.

"On Saturday last, the 24th inst., I visited the Jail Hospital, in company with Dr. Esdaile, for the purpose of seeing a prisoner awakened out of the mesmeric trance, who had been suffering for some time with an inflamed eye. Upon our arrival the man was awake, and no further experiment could therefore be tried with this patient. Another, however, immediately presented himself, who had never been subjected to the mesmeric influence before, and whom, I believe, the doctor had never seen. He had been suffering much for some days from severe pains in the head and face; though not at that moment in pain, it was thought advisable to try the effects of Mesmerism as a *preventive*. The manipulations were immediately commenced, and in seven minutes the man was in a cataleptic state. We tried various means to test the intensity of the trance: his limbs rigidly maintained themselves in any posture in which Dr. Esdaile chose to place them; and at last he was raised upon his feet; his back being slightly bent, his arms stretched over head, which was drooping upon his shoulder, and he remained fixed in this constrained position for some time, without exhibiting any symptoms of consciousness, or uneasiness. After a few minutes he was left to his deep repose, reclined upon the ground; and I understand that, since this first trial, he has never had the slightest return of the pains of which he previously complained: we were much astonished at the phenomena exhibited on this occasion; the limbs being so extraordinarily supple, and at the same time capable of being so rigidly fixed in any position, at the will of the operator. (Signed) F. FISHER."

"*Chinsurah, May 29th*, 1845."

May 25th.—Nazir Mahomed, entranced yesterday for conjunctivitis, has slept well all night. There is no pain in the head; very slight uneasiness about the eye: no watering. The zone of blood-vessels around the cornea is gone, and the inflammation is reduced from the vivid redness of the acute stage to the dull, brick-red colour of the chronic state. He can now see very well with the inflamed eye.

I put him on a high stool before me, and desired him to tell me when he became sleepy, but he had not time to do so, as I left him sitting entranced in five minutes: this was done with the idea of lessening the determination of blood to the head. I then proceeded to my usual business in Chinsurah, and was there introduced to Mr. M'Questen, the dentist, who was on a professional visit at the house of one of my patients. As he expressed a great desire to see some of my Mesmeric cases, I said that he had better take the present opportunity, as I had left a man entranced, and hoped to find him so on my return, and that others were undergoing the process at the Charity Hospital, but I knew not with what results.

The lady and gentleman of the house, hereupon, suddenly resolved to go, too; and the expedition gave rise to a little episode, which I have the pleasure of introducing here, by permission.

We returned to the Jail Hospital, after I had been absent an hour, and found the man sitting precisely as I had left him, and his body colder than natural. The influence was now nearly worn out (partly, no doubt, by the exhausting position,) and he awoke soon after our arrival. He said that the eye was still farther improved, and it looked so. I consider the case terminated. It was evident, to the most unpractised eye, that inflammation was incompatible with such a state of the system.

But a man sitting on a high stool for an hour without knowing it, was not enough to satisfy the curiosity and unbelief of my lady visitor. Her theory was, that I must be "*Angelus aut Diabolus,*" to be permitted to do such things; and as both hypothesis had their difficulties, she took refuge in an unapproachable unbelief. This to me was a singular mental phenomenon, and I determined to experiment upon her mind through her own senses (as she would not believe her husband even,) and to observe the effects. The man entranced for hemicrania yesterday was sent for, and put upon the stool. The gentlemen pulled out their watches, and in three minutes he was as insensible to life as the stool on which he sat. He was now put through all the amazing postures already described, and his friends were called in to awake him, but all to no purpose, till I came to their aid, when he awoke with a violent start, and look of alarm; and, on being questioned, said that he had gone to sleep of his own accord.

My honoured visitor had now evidently some difficulty in collecting her senses, and kept exclaiming,—"It's impossible! it can't be! I *won't* believe it; it's all a trick!" I replied, "If you will be good enough to go to the other hospital, I shall, perhaps, be able to show you more tricks of the same kind."

Having entered the "Blue Chamber," she was resolved to see its mysteries, and the party proceeded. I had ordered a man to be mesmerised in the morning, to have a tooth taken out; and, on reaching the Charity Hospital, had the satisfaction to find him entranced, and begged Mr. Mc'Questen to give him the benefit of his skill. This he declined; and I extracted the tooth before him, without awaking the man, and presented it to the lady as a mesmeric "souvenir." Seeing a collection of matter near the ear, I also made an incision into the swelling before he awoke. On coming to his senses he said that he felt as if an ant had bit him while he was asleep.

I had now the gratification, rarely granted to first believers,—of living to see the triumph of the truth. My fair infidel frankly gave up the "diabolic theory;" and although she could not yet adopt the angelic one in my favour, yet she was convinced that, instead of being in league with the evil power, I was a highly favoured individual, and congratulated me on my new powers of doing good. At parting I took the liberty to hint, in the most respectful manner, that there was something still more wonderful to me than Mesmerism; and that was, the extent of human incredulity on the subject.

June 6th.—I was called at 8 o'clock last night, to see the wife of Baboo Essanchunder Ghosaul, deputy-magistrate of Hooghly. I found her in dreadful convulsions; she was speechless, and suffering from a constriction in the throat, that threatened to suffocate her every minute; and she constantly beat, or pointed at the part. At one moment her body was perfectly rigid, and in another it was bent back like a bow, till she rested on the back of her head and heels only. I never saw such convulsions except in Tetanus and Hydrophobia, and all I knew of the resources of medicine was useless; for how could she take physic when she could not take breath! I therefore had recourse to my new solvent power, and, after nearly an hour's hard work, I left her asleep, and catalepsed.

July 1st.—She has had no return of the fit. This is the lady for whose relief the conjurer was sent, but came too late.

June 26th.—Alunga, aged 24; she has slight contractions of both elbow-joints, from rheumatism, with acute pain on pressing the ulnar nerve at the elbow. At first, she did not bear much handling without awaking; but, on being left alone, the trance deepened, and she permitted me to work her joints like door hinges, and extend them to the natural degree, without awaking. One arm was much freer after the first trance and extension, and there was no pain.

June 27th.—Complains of considerable pain in her left arm to-day, and the nerve at the elbow is very tender. I passed my fingers along the course of the nerve for a few minutes, which removed the pain, and allowed her to extend the arm: I then held my fingers before her eyes for a few seconds, and she fell into my arms insensible.

July 3rd.—This woman's pains fly about, but I can chase them away from any part by holding my fingers over it for a short time. She came limping up to me to-day, to have the pain taken out of her "tendo Achillis;" and this I did by passing my fingers over the pained part. I then grasped it firmly: she felt no pain, and by words and looks expressed the utmost astonishment and delight. This woman's sensibility is such, that I, or any one, can now make her delirious by merely looking at her for five minutes; but more of this hereafter.

Aug. 18th.—I requested Dr. Bedford to satisfy himself if the woman Alunga had pain in any part of her body. On being asked, she said there was acute pain in one heel; and Dr. B. spent a long time in testing the reality of its existence. He at last said that he was convinced there was considerable pain in that spot. I then passed my fingers over the part for a minute, and grasped the heel as firmly as I could, and she declared the pain had vanished; and Dr. B. allowed that it had. He then looked at her steadily, and in a few minutes developed the mesmeric delirium, and desire to sleep-walk, always produced in this woman, if the influence is not quickly concentrated upon her: the other symptoms, tremor of the eyelids, inability to open them when closed, and the mesmeric trance, all followed in due course.

July 4th.—Dookee, a shop-keeper. For several months has had a constant feeling of insects crawling about his face and scalp, and it often extends to the whole body; his eyes wink and water constantly. He was mesmerised for an hour, and then got a dose of mesmerised water. He soon after complained of general agitation, and feeling of alarm at the heart, and then slept a little. On leaving the hospital the sense of formication had entirely disappeared, and he did not wink more than was natural: he has not returned.

July 13th.—Four men and one woman were entranced to-day.

No. 1. for Lumbago.

No. 2. for Sciatica.

No. 3. for pain in the course of the crural nerve.

No. 4. for Syphilitic rheumatism.

No. 5. ditto.

They were all subdued by the usual manipulations, assisted by the breath.

After the first day the trance was induced in them all, by

giving mesmerised water daily, till the 17th: on which day the three with neuralgic pains were dismissed cured; the syphilitic cases were not benefitted, as might be expected, the constitutional specific disease being still in operation: the local pains were eased, however, and sleep procured: no small matter in such cases.

July 29th.—Sustee Ram, a bearer; aged 30. He became paralytic in his left arm, twelve days ago, during the night: he cannot raise it higher than his navel; there is pain under the capula; and he has slept very little since the attack:—to be mesmerised daily, for half-an-hour.

July 30th.—Slept all night, can raise his arm to his breast, head, spine, shoulder, and arm:—to be mesmerised daily.

July 31st.—Slept yesterday, immediately after being mesmerised, and all night: can touch the opposite shoulder and his forehead to-day.

Aug. 15th.—Has improved daily: usually sleeps after the process, and well at night.

Aug. 25th.—Can hold his arm perpendicular, and has considerable command over it.

Sept. 8th.—Can clap his hands above his head, strikes out well with the left arm, and squeezes my hand with considerable force. Discharged at his own request, being fit for work.

The next case I should never have taken in hand, if new hopes had not been infused into me by the evident effects of Mesmerism on the nervous system.

Aug. 9th.—Geeois, a husbandman; aged 22. A man of large frame, and in good condition. There is complete palsy of the whole of the left side; the arm can only be separated from the side for a few inches. He has taken mercury six times, in four years, for rheumatism: the paralysis began four months ago, and he has been three months in his present state:—to be mesmerised for half an hour daily.

Aug. 18th.—He sometimes goes to sleep during the process, and generally sleeps for two hours after it: he can raise his arm more, and there is a little resistance on the left side, on walking between two persons.

Aug. 20th.—He began to walk a little with a stick to-day.

Aug. 25th.—Improves daily; there is more command over the diseased side; the leg is stronger, and he raises the arm higher: he walked to the end of the room to-day, with the help of a stick only.

Sept. 8th.—Much better; walks across the compound, with the aid of a stick; arm also improving.

Sept. 20th.—He has discarded his stick, and crosses the compound unaided.

Sept. 25th.—Daily improving; he can hold his arm nearly perpendicular: there is every prospect of his recovering, and he was allowed to go home, with orders to his friends to mesmerise him daily, in the way they had witnessed.

Dec. 10th.—Horo, a Hindoo woman; aged 28. She has suffered for three years from *tic-doloureux* in the right eyebrow and temple, especially in the cold weather: it is very intense now, and comes on at 6 A. M., remaining till 2 P. M.—to be mesmerised. I returned after an hour, and found her asleep: she awoke soon after, and said there was no pain whatever in the part now, and that "it was cold as water."

Jan. 8th.—She has *had no return of pain.*

Dec. 14th.—Podo, a Hindoo woman, a beggar; aged 40. She has been a cripple for a year and a half, from rheumatism in her shoulders and knees: there is much tenderness about the joints, and her knees are so weak that she cannot sit with her hams bent, and is obliged to ease herself standing, and she cannot rise from the ground without pushing herself up with her hands:—to be mesmerised an hour daily.

Dec. 16th.—Slept half an hour after the process to-day.

Dec. 17th.—Feels much better.

Dec. 18th.—Slept an hour to-day; the pain about the joints is much less; she can rise from the ground without aid, and walks much more freely.

Dec. 19th.—Says she has no pain, and is quite well: dismissed cured, at her own request.

Mesmerism, like other powerful natural agents, is not only a remedy, but becomes a formidable disease when pushed far, and deeply rooted in the constitution; and a knowledge of this is the key to a variety of anomalous phenomena,—mesmeric in their origin, but not directly produced by it at the time, and which give rise to absurd charges of imposture, delusion, &c., from persons totally ignorant of the subject. These are, in fact, the secondary or constitutional symptoms of the primary disease—Mesmerism,—which has contaminated the nervous system, and predisposed it to take on the Mesmeric action whenever it is deranged, especially by any thing having reference to the processes by which it was first developed in the system.

In this respect, Mesmerism very closely resembles Hysteria, which, however primarily induced, is apt to recur on any agitation of the body or mind, more particularly if it is in any way associated with the first disturbing cause; and they both correspond, in each being sometimes *voluntarily* producible. Every one knows how a *genuine* fit of hysterics can be *willed* on, and that often there can be no doubt of the *reality* of the exhibition; and, in like manner, some persons can *will* on somnambulism and the other Mesmeric symptoms, the reality of which are indisputable. To an experienced person, the springing up of true Mesmeric phenomena, without the usual exciting cause, is a moral demonstration that the system has been previously revolutionized by Mesmerism. The nervous centres having become morbidly sensitive by the action of this great nervous excitant, every shock of the nerves, especially if connected with Mesmerism, is exhibited in the shape of abnormal mesmeric symptoms.

The eye of the hunter can tell by the foot-prints the kind of animal that has gone before: from the shadow we can guess the semblance of the substance; and, in like manner, the qualified observer, when he sees pseudo-mesmeric appearances, at once says, the Mesmerist has been here before me—*ex pede Herculem.*

It is high time that the public should be disabused of many erroneous impressions regarding the finer phenomena of Mesmerism, which have been sedulously propagated by medical men even, affectedly impartial, but, in reality, labouring under intense prejudice, and profound ignorance of the subject.

It is of no consequence to the community whether it is misled by the ignorance or dishonesty of those who set themselves up as leaders of public opinion; the offence against truth, the injury done to the public, and the injustice to those who have practically studied the question, and declared what they know to be true, careless whom it may displease, are equally great. It is a common thing for Doctors, who have never seen or thought of Mesmerism, to step forward to enlighten the public, and expose the "humbug." They have heard of "Mesmeric coma," and that, under its influence, the most severe surgical operations can be performed without pain; and they thereupon exact *total insensibility* into their *experimentum crucis* of the truth of Mesmerism; and if any unfortunate Mesmeric wight, having a vulnerable point in his "tendo Achillis" even, should fall under their observation, he is denounced as a hardened and determined impostor, and his physician exposed as a quack, or charitably allowed to be, perhaps, only a fool.

Nothing short of the extinction of life will satisfy these discriminating observers: physiological revolutions in the system—altered bearing—changed expression in features and voice—the approach and advance of sleep—the extinction of some senses—and the preservation or exaltation of others, are all not only lost upon such philosophers, but are, one and all, "confirmations, strong as Holy Writ," of the existence of imposture! Such is the procrustean bed to which the anti-mesmerists bind down Nature in this most varied and wonderful display of her powers. If the body of their venerable mother be longer than her unnatural children, the Doctors, wish it, they mercilessly amputate the offending members: if shorter, she is pulled and stretched by pulleys, *secundem artem,* to the length prescribed. A dispassionate and candid judge of this description (the wolf judging the lamb) is perhaps invited by a medical Mesmerist to satisfy himself by ocular demonstration in his hospitals, since nothing short of this can affect his understanding; and the Mesmeric guest commences his course of practical experiment by tossing and goring the patients (fortunately generally insensible) like a mad bull; his only thought being how to kill two at a blow; and because he has been compelled to develop all the Mesmeric phenomena *himself,* he revenges himself by declaring it to be all a miserable imposture and delusion: passion is the same all over the world, and it is easier to instruct ignorance than pride.

But I am anxious that the public should know what Mesmerism really is, in order that they may know it when it comes before them, and be no longer deluded by prejudiced, ignorant, or interested *quasi* descriptions of it. Abundant examples of its acute, and extreme effects on the system will be found in these pages, as well as many of the intermediate phases, and each, to the discriminating observer, is distinctive and characteristic of an unusual condition of the body. The *involuntary* quivering of the eyelids, and the spasmodic closing of the eye, in persons a minute before wide awake, and resisting, perhaps;—the extinction of one or more of the organs of sense, which we saw in full activity but a moment ago;—the eye turned up so that the white can only be seen, or staring wide open, fixed and insensible to light;—sleep walking,—delirium,—convulsions,—

catalepsy, in persons not subject to these affections till they were subjected to the mesmeric processes;—is not any one of these induced symptoms as clearly the effect of some constraining influence as the production of insensibility? They are all links of the same chain, and in some patients can all be beautifully exhibited in sequence and connection, from the quivering of an eyelash to the most intense coma.

Another anti-mesmerist, who to save appearances has condescended to look at certain of the mesmeric phenomena, says, on seeing their reality:—"There is no use in denying the extraordinary condition these people are reduced to; but the whole secret of the matter is that they are a set of poor hysterical wretches, and I will show you that I can mesmerise them as well as you, by *doing nothing*." The enterprising experimentalist proceeds to redeem his pledge, and actually succeeds, to his great delight and the mystification of the public, in disproving the truth of the axiom, "*ex nihilo nihil fit*,"—for he produces a serious disease, hysteria, by the compelling power of *nothing!* Upon this, the obstructives congratulate each other, and call upon the public to put down the naked humbug. Would not the public suppose that this mesmerising *by nothing* was an ingenious and original experiment of the anti-mesmeric school of philosophy? And yet the truth is, that they were taught their favourite trick by the *Mesmerists;* who have not only declared, that this can be done, but that it is a *natural consequence* of their proceedings, if carried to a certain extent. It is often very difficult, and laborious, to excite the mesmeric action in the constitution; but being once excited, a very slight recurrence to the original processes will bring on the paroxysm in all its first intensity, and if the excitement of the nervous system is kept up by frequent mesmerising, it takes on an independent diseased action, obeying constitutional laws which we do not understand: we, in fact, have inoculated the system with a nervous disease which often acts *spontaneously,* especially on any reference to the primary exciting cause; and at this stage the *candid medical observer* steps in, and demands the applause of an admiring and confounded world, for having done with "nothing," what had cost his stupid mesmeric brother so much trouble to effect.

It is hardly credible that Dr. Elliotson had expressly said, and that our candid philosophers knew it:—"At length there is sometimes such sensibility, that almost any thing will induce sleep; indeed, no process at last may be requisite to produce the effect. I have three patients, whom I was originally some weeks in sending to sleep, though I gave each half an hour daily of manipulations, and gazing; but who now go to sleep on my merely raising my hand, or looking at them when they are prepared to expect sleep. I told each of them that, if she sat still, I would mesmerise her in the next room through the door. I retired, shut the door behind me, *did nothing*, but walked into a further room, turned back, and found her asleep: so with the other two in succession. While I did this, I thought as little of them as possible, and busied myself with any thing to distract my attention."—Mesmerists in all parts of the world have stated the same fact, and I can bear the most ample testimony to its truth.

What candid mind, after considering this explanation, will regard "mesmerising by nothing," as a demonstration of the imposture of Mesmerism?

I was explaining the *mesmeric disease* (for such it has become, at this stage) to a party of gentlemen, the other day, and while speaking, a man anticipated my intention to mesmerise him "by nothing," by becoming intensely entranced on the spot, when I was not regarding him. The gentlemen, and Dr. Scott among them, used every means to ascertain his condition, and were as well convinced that he had lost his senses, as that they were in possession of theirs:—in fact, although the paroxysm was spontaneous, he would have borne a severe surgical operation without feeling it. I went to the hospital to-day (8th Dec. 1845) after writing the last line, and had there the pleasure of meeting Dr. Behn, Professor of Anatomy and Physiology in the University of Kiel, Mr. Kiellerup, Naturalist, and Mr. Blyth, Curator of the Asiatic Society's museum: the two former gentlemen are attached to the Danish frigate, now here on a political and scientific mission. As all three were observers of nature by profession, I thought it a good opportunity to correct my own impressions by theirs, if different from mine, and therefore submitted to their notice cases of direct and indirect Mesmerism. A man was brought before us with an enlarged and tender testis, and of the latter point Dr. Behn satisfied himself and friends, by pressing the part—there could be no mistake about it. I then, by the hands and breath, mesmerised him, standing before me, till he could not open his eyes, and the sensibility of the skin had disappeared. Dr. Behn then used any degree of pressure he chose to apply to the tender part, and the man's face was as placid as a statue of Somnus; every means was used to ascertain the state of the skin and the organs of sense, and it was clear that the ear was the only organ that transmitted any sensation to the brain, and this only of *sound;* when water was squirted suddenly into his ear, he said that he felt nothing, and on waking, he was surprised to find his face wet. I also converted him into a somnambulist, that the gentlemen might at once have before them as many as possible of the genuine mesmeric phenomena. Another man was then brought; and on asking him about his health, he said that he was feverish and had a severe pain in the side. This was evidently the case; for Dr. Behn pressed between the ribs, and found the intercostal spaces exceedingly tender. I then put him in a corner of the room, and bid him sleep: in less than five minutes he was asleep, could not turn round, or open his eyes, catalepsy was established, and all sensibility had disappeared; as Dr. Behn ascertained by now pressing between the ribs to any degree he pleased;—and not only so, the whole chest was seen to be catalepsed and immovable. His eyelids were forced open, and the white of the eye could only be seen. The moment he awoke, Dr. Behn again made pressure on the intercostal spaces, and he showed immediate and acute suffering.—In a word, the spontaneous mesmeric condition differed in no particular from that induced by the direct application of the mesmeric influence, and my visitors seemed to be perfectly satisfied of the reality of the symptoms in both states.

It would be tedious to dwell on this point farther, and I hope enough has been said to convince the public that, in general, when people are said to have been mesmerised "by nothing," it is a certain proof that *something* has pre-disposed to this, and we know nothing that can do this but *Mesmerism.* It is hardly worth while to dispute about names; and if it is allowed that I can cure nervous headaches, and perform painless surgical operations by hysteria, call the process hysteric or mesmeric—I care not.

But after all, there *is* a satisfaction in calling things by their right names, and I cannot possibly see how hysteria has got into my hospitals, where I never saw it before—coolies and felons not being at all nervous subjects. I have, therefore, generated a new disease among my patients by *nothing,* or by using the mesmeric processes. Which is the more likely, I leave my readers to decide. As natural hysteria may be supposed to be more powerful than the imitation, I shall look with impatience for the announcement, in "The Morning Post," that Mrs. Freak has been cured of her nervous headaches by the skilful application of hysteria, and Lady Tantrum has had her arm cut off when in a fit of hysterics, without knowing it. These should be easy feats for our fashionable physicians and surgeons, as they have the disease and antidote ready made to their hands; whereas, it cost me and my assistants great trouble to make the coolies and prisoners of Bengal hysterical, to the degree necessary to render them insensible to the loss of their members.

But seriously, if medical men wish to see and understand the effects of Mesmerism on the body, the natural and rational mode of proceeding is to attempt to develop them in the persons of their own patients; and if they will take a tithe of the trouble I have been at, I can promise them very general success. The finest, as well as the most striking phenomena will then be equally diagnostic to their practised eyes, and their understandings will be left clear, and free to study and imitate the curative processes of Nature, undisturbed by doubts and suspicions regarding the powers of observation and the honesty of others.

CHAPTER VII.

Mesmerism in Surgery.—Journal of Practical Mesmerism.—Mesmeric Trance: A Leg straightened in; Colic cured by; Penis amputated in; Arm straightened in; Arm amputated in; Breast cut off in; Abscess opened in; Heel flayed in; Tooth extracted in; End of Thumb cut off in; Arm laid open in; Three Abscesses opened in; Sinus laid open in; Gum cut away in; Invasion of the waking by the sleeping State.—Mesmeric Trance: Hypertrophied Prepuce cut off in; Suppurating Pile in; Both great Toe Nails cut out in; Knee straightened in; Ulcer on Temple burned with Muriatic Acid in; Seton introduced, &c. in; Tumour in Groin removed in; Fungoid Sores pared off in; Scirrhus Testes extirpated in; Cataract operated on in; Malignant Disease of Testes extirpated in; Unhealthy Sore pared in; Hypertrophied Prepuce cut off in; Pain extinguished by; Return on awaking; Amputation of Penis in; Unhealthy Sores pared in; Two Operations for Hydrocele in.—Mesmerism alike favourable to the Operator and the Patient.

In Surgery, the benefits of Mesmerism are not confined to the extinction of pain during an operation, but are of the greatest general and particular advantage in the after-treatment of surgical diseases. The nerves and brain have not been shattered by bodily and mental anguish, which generally excites an irritative fever in the system, wasting the powers of life, and rousing local inflammation in the injured part; thereby often destroying all the hopes and precautions of the surgeon. In the mesmeric sleep, only the necessary local injury has been inflicted; and on awaking, the patient sometimes feels no pain whatever, and generally only a slight smarting in the wound; and the constitution sets about repairing the breach of substance quietly, and under the best possible circumstances; if local pains follow, they can be easily removed by topical manipulations; all which will be seen in the following

Journal of Practical Mesmerism.

April 20th.—Jeolal, my washerman, aged 35, has been eighteen months ill; first with dysentery, afterwards with rheumatic fever, in consequence of which his left knee is bent upon the thigh at a right angle.

I considered him to be a hopeless cripple. I mesmerised him to-day in a quarter of an hour. At first he supported his knee with both hands; but soon allowed me to remove them, and suspend them in the air. The leg was then gradually extended, and straightened to a considerable extent, without awaking him.

April 21st.—The process was repeated to-day, and more force used, which awoke him; the leg was still farther improved.

April 22d.—The pulley was used to-day, and very considerable power applied before he awoke. The muscular contraction is now nearly overcome, and the remaining stiffness of the knee seems to be from the tendons and ligaments about the joint, and will probably yield to mechanical extension, by exercise.

May 11th.—He can now walk without a stick, but the fibrous contractions give way slowly. I am convinced that direct force might have torn the muscles of the thigh, but could not have relaxed them.

June 22d.—His leg is now quite straight, and the knee flexible; he has got a violent colic, and when speaking to me fell down in a fainting state.—Ordered to be mesmerised.

June 23d.—He slept for an hour, and awoke much relieved yesterday; but a paroxysm returned last night, and still continues.—Repeat the Mesmerism.

June 24th.—He remained three hours in the mesmeric sleep yesterday, and awoke quite well, and continues so. His leg is now quite strong, and he has returned to his work.

May 12th.—Buxoo, a Khitmatgan. There is a fistulous opening in the urethra under the glans penis, which is sloughing, and requires to be amputated. I desired him to be mesmerised, and returned in an hour. I found him asleep, and when looking at him, he suddenly opened his eyes, but immediately went to sleep again, and in five minutes after I cut off the glans, without awaking him. He awoke soon after, and said it was from fear, not pain.

April 20th, 11 o'clock, A. M.—Kangalee, a peasant; aged 20, weak, and ill nourished. He had a fever four years ago, after which sores broke out in different parts of his body, and have left large cicatrices like burns. There is one about the left elbow joint, which has been permanently contracted to nearly a right angle, for seven months. He was catalepsed in twenty minutes; a bottle was then put under his elbow for a fulcrum, and the arm was gradually extended by depressing the hand. He moved a little, and the muscles contracted occasionally, but soon melted as it were, under my hand, and I left him, with his arm perfectly straight, extended in the air and still asleep.—Two o'clock, P. M. He awoke half an hour ago. Sees his arm is straight, knows not how it was done, has no pain, and can move it freely.

May 2d.—He pulls the punkah daily with his left arm, for exercise.

June 14th.—Dismissed cured.

May 5th.—Rantoonee Buttachangie, a Brahmin; aged 40. There is a prodigious Fungus hæmatodes protruding from the left elbow-joint. A swelling took place at the joint when he was five years old, and has gone on increasing gradually, but the skin remained entire till an incision was made by a native doctor, twelve days ago, when the bloody mass started through the integuments. It exactly resembles the contents of an old aneurism; the structure of the fungus having been broken up by the actual cautery applied to it all over, in order to stop the bleeding: it was a frightful mass. I desired him to be carefully mesmerised, and went to Chinsurah, to consult with Dr. Elton, in charge of the troops there. We returned to the hospital together, and found him in a profound sleep, and decided to take the arm off instantly. It was removed, without his moving or complaining, and Dr. Elton assured me that his countenance had never changed. He awoke immediately after the limb was off, and declared, again and again, that he was aware of nothing having been done to him till he awoke and saw his arm was gone; and he then saw Dr. Elton for the first time.

May 13th.—Is doing well.

May 16th.—He complains of pain in the stump to-day.—To be mesmerised.

May 17th.—He was easily put to sleep yesterday, and slept

for three hours; was free from pain when he awoke, and continues so.

May 11th.—Meeroolla, a policeman; aged 28, strong and healthy looking. He has got a fatty tumour of the right mamma, which he begged me to remove to-day. I desired him to lie down, and let me carefully examine it, and commenced mesmerising him. In ten minutes he was fast asleep; in five minutes more I transfixed the tumour with a hook, drew it up off the muscles, and cut it out, without disturbing him in the least, and he did not awake till half an hour afterwards. He declares that he felt no pain till he awoke, and remembers nothing after my hands were placed on his stomach, which was in about five minutes from the commencement.

May 11th.—Podoo, a young Hindoo woman, has a swelling over the false ribs of the right side, requiring an incision to be made in it. I desired the compounder to mesmerise her, while I was engaged with the last patient, and she was ready before I was: a deep incision, an inch long, was made into the swelling, without awaking her, and I left her sleeping.

May 14th.—Maduh, a healthy-looking coolie; aged 30. I saw him for the first time to-day, at 11 o'clock. He has got a sore on the heel, of two years' standing; the skin is half an inch thick, separated from the subjacent parts all round, and requires to be removed.—To be mesmerised. I went on to Chinsurah, where I had the pleasure to be introduced to the Reverend Mr. Banergie, who is there on a visit, and who begged me to show him a person under the mesmeric influence. I replied that I disapproved of experimenting with so formidable a power, to gratify mere curiosity; but I had left a man under the process, and that if he would go to the hospital, on chance, he might possibly be gratified. I returned to the hospital after an hour, and there found the Reverend Mr. Fisher, Mr. Banergie, and Mr. Money, the collector. The patient was asleep, and I immediately commenced dissecting the thickened skin from the plantar fascia, which was very difficult, owing to its thickness and hardness. It almost resembled a horse's hoof, and removal must have been very painful under ordinary circumstances. He was completely insensible to the pain, however, and remained asleep a quarter of an hour after I had finished.

Mr. Banergie then questioned him, in Bengalee, regarding

his feelings, and he protested that he felt nothing till he awoke. Many of the patients, already mentioned, being still in hospital, Mr. Banergie examined them in Bengalee, and in no instance did their accounts vary from what I had related.

May 26th.—Ram Dass, a large robust man, has a supernumerary tooth between the eye-tooth, and the first grinder, growing horizontally into his mouth, and causing him great annoyance. I entranced him in a quarter of an hour, lying on a mattress on the table, and proceeded to open his jaws. It cost me some trouble to relax the temporal muscles, and I had to proceed cautiously, as he did not appear to be under the extreme influence of the mesmeric power. From its position, it was difficult to lay hold of the tooth, but it was at last grasped, and extracted. He moved, and moaned a little, but I soon tranquillised him again, and he did not awake till almost suffocated by the blood. He declared he awoke from this cause, and not from pain.

May 29th.—Sibehurn Sing, a young robust man, had his thumb nearly cut through by a sword, fourteen days ago. An attempt was made to unite it, but failed; and the point of the finger would be a nuisance if kept. In ten minutes I made him insensible, and cut off the end of the thumb without awaking him. He soon after quietly opened his eyes, and I asked him:—"Have you been asleep?" "Yes." "Have you any pain?" "No." "Has any thing hurt you to-day?" "No." "Do you wish your nail cut off?" "Yes." "Look at it." He did so, looked confounded, and exclaimed, "It's gone!" "Who did it?" "God knows." "How did it happen, has it fallen off itself?" "I can't tell—I know nothing about it."

May 30th.—Modoomohun Ray, a fine boy, 12 years old, was brought to the hospital, fourteen days ago, with a compound fracture of both bones of the forearm, and my assistants had several times tried to mesmerise him, in the hope of assuaging the pain, but without success. Matter has formed, and the wound must be enlarged, upwards and downwards. As he was apprehensive, I put a piece of wet cloth over his eyes, and went on with my affairs, telling him that it would cool his brain. The people were all dismissed, and approaching him unobserved, I succeeded in entrancing him in ten minutes, and laid open the arm without disturbing him. I returned after three hours, and found him still sleeping. On awaking, he said the pain was much less, and that no one had hurt him that day.

June 2d.—Gungaram Dass, a prisoner, was injured, ten days ago, by some rubbish falling on him, and in consequence three large abscesses have formed at the elbow, wrist, and ankle, which require to be opened. I subdued him in a few minutes, opened the abscesses, and left him sleeping. On my return, after two hours, he had just awoke, and I found him sitting up looking at his wounds. I asked him how the pus had escaped, since I saw him in the morning? He could not tell. Of its own accord? He supposed so. Had any one cut or hurt him to-day? No one.

June 16th.—Toorab, a peasant, aged 30, of a rickety constitution, has a sinus, six inches in length, under the pectoral muscle, of seven months' standing. We have not been able to close it by any means, and it is necessary to lay it open. He was entranced by one of my assistants, and I laid the whole of the diseased tract open without his knowing it, and left him sleeping.

June 15th.—He awoke soon after I left him, and on awaking, asked where the blood had come from? He has hardly had any pain in the wound, and has no recollection of being disturbed in his sleep yesterday.

July 9th.—Mrs. Clermont is suffering from one of her wisdom teeth; half of it has come through, but the rest is covered with the indurated and ulcerated gum. I explained that the source of the irritation must be removed, by cutting away the offending gum.

July 10th.—I entranced her to-day, sitting on a couch, in the presence of her husband and his sister; laid her back and cut away the gum without awaking her, and left her sleeping.

July 11th.—This is a very interesting case, as it shows the invasion of the waking by the sleeping state. Mrs. C., on awaking yesterday, arose as if from common sleep, and went to adjust her hair in the glass, when she saw blood about her mouth, and this first attracted her attention to the tooth; she thought the gum had burst, and was still expecting me to call. For, strange to say, she had no recollection of having seen me that day, nor of what happened for half an hour before I put her to sleep. The incidents, her husband informed me, that occurred during this time were these:—She received letters from the postman, and paid for them; a lady came to visit her; and then I arrived, and sat conversing with them a short time. After seeing the lady to her carriage, I returned and mesmerised her:—all these occurrences were blotted from her mind. She feels quite well, and awoke much refreshed. If such inroads are made into the regions of sense, at one sitting, the effect of frequent unnecessary experiments may be guessed at in such sensitive subjects as this lady; and this is the power trifled with, and made a show of for money!*

July 17th.—To-day, in the presence of Mr. Davidson, commissioner of the district, and Mr. Alexander, Registrar to the Board of Revenue (who have requested me to name them as witnesses,) I operated on a man for hypertrophy of the prepuce, without awaking him. After letting him sleep some time, I asked the gentlemen if I should awake him, and at their desire, did so in a moment, by blowing in his eyes. He was restored at once to full consciousness, and Mr. Davidson remarked, "I wish Doctor —— was here, who says you do this by opium." My visitors, understanding Bengalee, asked him if any one had hurt him to-day. He said, "No." If he would like his disease to be

*While in London, arranging for the publication of this work, I had the pleasure of being introduced to Dr. Elliotson, under whose guidance I mesmerised two females, although I had never before seen Mesmerism, or attempted to practise it. These women being accustomed to be mesmerised, I was not surprised at my success; but an event which happened a few days afterwards, astonished both myself and the friends who witnessed the occurrence. At an evening party I met a young gentleman from Oxford, who requested me to mesmerise him. He had never seen Mesmerism; and yet, in one minute, his eyes closed under my manipulations, and in less than three minutes he was fast asleep. Being diffident in my own powers, I de-mesmerised him as speedily as possible. He thus described his sensations: "The moment you pointed your fingers at me, I felt uncomfortable. I dared not meet your gaze; a sensation of heat, resembling a stream of electricity, commenced at my forehead and followed the course of your hands, down to the pit of my stomach. I could not open my eyes. I knew I was sitting on a chair before you, and the last idea in my mind, before falling fast asleep, was this—Shall I ever be allowed to rise again?"

This fact seems to prove that the power of mesmerising, and of being mesmerised, is more general in this country than is commonly supposed.—Editor.

removed? He answered, that he would thank God if any one would do so. He was then desired to sit up, and his cloth removed; when, seeing his nuisance was gone, he fell back with an exclamation of wonder and gratitude.

July 25th.—Buggabuttee, a Hindoo woman, aged 40, has been troubled with a suppurating pile, as big as the end of my thumb. She was mesmerised at eleven o'clock, and at twelve I cut off the tumour, and though she moved and moaned, on awaking half an hour after, did not know that any thing had been done to her.

Aug. 4th.—Sona, a Hindoo woman; 25 years old. Both nails of the great toes are destroyed to the roots, by the combined effects of syphilis and mercury, and their place is filled with a fungoid ulcer. She was mesmerised at twelve o'clock, and at half past one P. M., I dissected out the entire root of one nail, without awaking her: her left hand and arm trembled only, and this was subdued in a few minutes, by her hand being held in mine.—Left her sleeping.

Aug. 5th.—Again entranced, and I cut out the other nail without annoying her. On neither occasion has she had any pain on awaking.

Aug. 6th.—Golam Hassein. His knee has been contracted to a considerable extent for two months, from rheumatism. He was mesmerised for the first time at eleven o'clock, and I made his leg straight at one o'clock, the new ligamentous adhesions were felt, and heard, cracking under my hands.—He felt no pain on awaking.

Aug. 8th.—Gendo, a Hindoo woman; aged 50. There is a large sloughing ulcer, covering all her right temple. She was mesmerised at ten o'clock A. M.; and at half past eleven, I freely applied muriatic acid to the whole sore, without her showing any sensibility. She awoke twenty minutes after, and knew nothing about it.

Aug. 9th.—Parbuttie, an elderly Hindoo woman, has a sinus extending from the inner ankle, under the calf, to the outer side of the leg near the knee, which is contracted by a dense cicatrix running two thirds round the joint, and involving the hamstrings: the knee has been in this state for ten years. Being put to sleep, a counter opening was made in the leg, and a seton run through the leg, without her feeling it. I then leant all my weight on the knee, and succeeded in extending it a little, but the diseased structures would yield no farther. A heavier and stronger gentleman then applied all his power, and effected a little more, but it was evident that no force short of breaking the limb could straighten it. But it was equally certain, that any common muscular or ligamentous contraction must have yielded on the spot.—The woman continued to sleep for hours after.

Aug. 23d.—Napaul Bagdy, a husbandman, has a singular fungoid mass in the right groin; it is the size of a small cauliflower, and like it in appearance, the surface being whitish from sloughing. It spreads from a peduncle in the abdominal ring, and bleeds much when handled. His father says that, at his birth, there was only one testis in the scrotum, and no trace of the other was seen till he was six months old, when a swelling appeared in the groin. This gradually increased till his twelfth year, but was not painful or inconvenient. About this time he was attacked with fever, attended with increased sensibility and increase of size in the tumour, and the paroxysms came on twice a month, up to June last, when he applied to a barber-surgeon, who used means *to ripen* the swelling. In the course of a few days it was punctured, and blood only followed. The opening was plugged as well as possible with a candle covered with cloth smeared with some ointment, but in a few days this came out, and the following day, a fungus shot out of the wound, and daily increased to its present size. It is now a very foul mass, its surface mortified and the crevices filled with maggots.

Aug. 26th.—He was mesmerised after two hours' trial, and the mass removed without his feeling it.

Aug. 31st.—Discharged at his own request—wound looking well.

Sept. 1st.—Raimgopal, a young Hindoo, has got a high syphilitic sore, about the size of half a lemon, on each side of his nates. He was entranced on the first trial; and in the presence of Dr. Ross and Dr. Sissmore, I turned him round like a log, and cut off both the excrescences level with the skin, then turned him back again, and left him sleeping. It is needless to say he did not feel it.

Oct. 8th.—Nazir, a peasant, aged 60, has suffered from enlarged and scirrhous testis for four years; the parts are as large as a child's head, and extirpation is necessary.—He was entranced after two hours to-day.

Oct. 10th.—He was mesmerised the second time, to-day, in the presence of Mr. Sutherland, Dr. Owen, the Reverend Mr. Bradbury, Major Riddle, Mr. Higgen, Mr. Muller, Mr. Graves, Messrs. Savigny, Mr. Calder, and Mr. Bartlett.

I removed the parts without his showing any sign of sensibility till the last artery was being tied: he then woke up, but went immediately to sleep again for half an hour, and on awaking, said that he was only conscious of a little pain when he awoke for a moment, and found me to be tying something. He was cheerful and talkative, and showed no signs of suffering or exhaustion in his countenance or manner, and said the pain in the wound was very trifling.

Nov. 20th.—Mohun Dass, a peasant; aged 55: has got a cataract in one eye. He was entranced on the first trial, and I broke down the lens in the presence of Major Smith of H. M.'s 9th Regt., without awaking him.

Nov. 21st.—There is much pain in the eye.—To be mesmerised, and leeches applied. He slept for two hours with the leeches on, and on awaking, the pain was nearly gone.

Nov. 26th.—Mahes Banergie, a Brahmin, aged 40, has got an enlarged testis, the size of a child's head; it is red, glistening, and very painful, and there is a scrotal hernia above it. He was entranced on the first trial, and I returned the gut into the abdomen, handling the inflamed part very rudely, without his showing the least sensibility. I then, in the presence of Captain D. L. Richardson, dissected out the diseased organ. The operation was tedious, as I had to carefully separate the mass from the hernial sack. He moved, as in an uneasy dream, but did not awake till we were tying the arteries, which were very numerous; he then said, that he had felt nothing till that moment. The muscular movements, sometimes seen, looked more like the contractions induced by cutting a recently dead animal, than the common contortions from pain; and I believe may be avoided by patience, as every trance seems to deepen the insensibility. I need not point out to the surgeon the advantage he would derive from the mesmeric trance, in reducing strangulated hernia, and spasmodic strictures of the urethra.

Nov. 30th.—Mahes, a peasant, aged 32, has got a deep ulcer of a year's standing, at the root of the penis, that penetrates under the pubes; the edges are callous, and prevent it healing. He was subdued in two hours on the first day, and in the presence of Dr. Tritton and a party of officers of the 71st Regiment N. I., I pared off the margins of the sore without his awaking. He awoke a few minutes after, said he had been asleep, and dreamt that some one had pulled him off the roof of a house, and declared that he felt *no pain whatever* at the moment of speaking. I thereupon proposed that he should allow me to cut him a very little, as it would facilitate the healing of the sore, but he would not hear of it. Dr. Tritton and the rest also joined their persuasions; but he implored us for the love of God to let him alone—he would rather die than be cut, that the proposal had already killed him, &c. He was desired to sit up, and his cloth removed; on seeing the altered state of things, he was greatly alarmed and puzzled, and on being shown the pieces of flesh, said they had certainly belonged to him before he went to sleep, and how I got hold of them he had no idea. As I found myself in the company of candid and dispassionate observers, I showed them Mesmerism in all its physical symptoms, whether directly or indirectly produced, and Dr. Tritton very kindly said at parting, that he was quite convinced of the *reality* of the symptoms from first to last, whether produced by *something*, or *nothing*, and that he now quite understood the "mesmeric disease," and said I was at liberty to say so, if I pleased.

Dec. 1st.—I had the pleasure of receiving a visit from the gentlemen engaged in the railway survey, consisting of Mr. Simms, Captain Western, Captain Boileau, Mr. Fraser, and Dr. Macauley. They found a man entranced, from whom I was about to remove a hypertrophied prepuce. As he appeared to be ready, I commenced at once; but seeing that he shrunk from the knife, without awaking, however, I desisted, and proposed to adjourn to the other hospital, saying that this man would probably be ready on our return. We accordingly went, and I requested Dr. Macauley to ascertain if a man brought before us had pain in his scrotum. He said there was no doubt; and the rest were satisfied that there was no mistake about it. I ordered him to be entranced before them, which was easily done, as he had been twice operated on for hydrocele, in the trance. I pulled him up, and set him on his feet sleeping, before the gentlemen, and begged them to deal with him as they pleased. He was catalepsed by them in the most painful attitudes, to which he was as indifferent as a man of clay; and Dr. Macauley now squeezed the painful part with as much effect as if the man had been a mummy. I stripped him naked; and when he awoke and found himself standing in the presence of gentlemen in this condition, his look of wonder and shame, if not natural, was most beautiful acting, and he certainly escaped being found out. As soon as he awoke, Dr. Macauley pressed the diseased part, and there could be no doubt about his feelings on the subject;—the pain was evidently instantaneous and acute. On returning to the Charity Hospital, I removed the enlarged cellular substance from the whole penis; the man did not shrink in the least from the knife, and slept a good while after the operation. On questioning him, he said that he had been put to sleep to be operated on; but as he was now awake, he would wish it to be put off till to-morrow. We then showed him the liberties that had been taken with him, and he recognised his property; but how it had changed owners he had no conception.

Dec. 21st.—Samoo, a weaver, has got a bad sloughing sore of the prepuce and glans, of a year's standing.—To be mesmerised.

Dec. 22d.—He was mesmerised for two hours yesterday, and slept an hour afterwards, apparently naturally. To-day I saw him after half an hour's mesmerising, when the trance was fully established, his whole body being rigid. As I had not time then, I left him, and returned in an hour, and found his body still stiff. I cut open and took off the prepuce; and finding the glans half eroded, I cut it off too. The man showed no sign of life; the body continued stiff, and the pulse natural. He awoke in half an hour afterwards, and did not discover that any thing had been done to him till he went to make water.

Dec. 29th.—Mahes, operated on last month. The sore is callous, and it will greatly advance his cure to have it pared.—To be mesmerised in my absence. I went on to Chinsurah, and there met the Rev. Mr. Cahusac, and the Rev. Mr. Mullins, who requested to see any mesmeric cases in hand. They returned with me to the hospital, and we found Mahes entranced. I pared the sore, and he did not awake till a quarter of an hour afterwards. Mr. Mullins, who speaks Bengalee, asked him if he had been disturbed in his sleep. He said "No;" and that the pain was not greater than before he went to sleep.

We found another man entranced, whose elbow had been dislocated for twenty days. I tried to reduce it, using all my force, but did not succeed; he moved uneasily, but did not awake till ten minutes after I had desisted, and then said that nothing had disturbed him.

Dec. 26th.—Goluck Seit, a prisoner, has got a hydrocele on each side. A young Hindoo subdued him to-day in ten minutes, on the first trial. When about to operate, I saw that he possessed a *consecrated nail,* on one of his little fingers; and knowing the value attached to this, I resolved to get possession of it, if possible, as a *moral* test of his being insensible, for he would as soon have cut a cow's throat and eaten a beefsteak as allowed me to cut off his nail, while in possession of his senses. It is a common practice with the Hindoos to vow their hair, beards, or nails to Shiva, the Destroyer, in the hope of averting his anger; and this man had consecrated his little finger-nail to Shiva Forakissore,—Forakissore, in this district, being a famous shrine of the god. I transferred the sacred excrescence to my pocket, without any remonstrance being made, and then performed the less formidable operation of withdrawing the water, and throwing in the injection, of which he knew nothing, on awaking two hours after. His only distress was the loss of his nail, and he spent hours in hunting for it, supposing that it had been broken off by accident.

Dec. 29th.—I entranced Goluck Seit to-day in five minutes; and in the presence of Mr. Cahusac and Mr. Mullins, operated on the other hydrocele, to which he was as indifferent as on the first occasion. But before putting him to sleep, I showed the gentlemen how painful was the side operated on three days ago; and yet, in five minutes after, he allowed me to squeeze his testicle to any extent, without exhibiting a vestige of uneasiness. I awoke him in half an hour, that Mr. Mullins might question him; and he said that he saw the water was gone, but how it had escaped he had no idea.

Dec. 30th.—Bungsee, operated on last month for a scrotal tumour. The wound, from his debilitated condition, is glazed and callous, and is wasting him with a useless discharge. It would greatly shorten his cure to pare the sore, and bring it together with deep sutures; but I could hardly bring myself to propose it to a person in his senses, as it would be as painful as the capital operation. Mesmerism, however, makes surgery pleasant to both parties; and having easily entranced him, I pared and shaped the sore very leisurely, (it was six inches long, by two deep,) inserted the deep sutures, and left him sleeping. He awoke after four hours.

Jan. 2d.—The sutures were taken out to-day, and the sore is adherent throughout.

This power of remedying any defect in the operation afterwards, without inflicting pain, is not one of the least advantages of Mesmerism.

CHAPTER VIII.

Hypertrophy of the Scrotum; different Causes of.—Elephantiasis endemic in Bengal and Lower Egypt; probable Causes of.—Example of Malarious Fever.—True Elephantiasis of the Scrotum.—Hypertrophy from Hydrocele; from Syphilis; Condition of the Organs involved; Mode of operating; Mismanagement by the Native Doctors; Number of Operations for Six Years previous to April, 1845; in the Mesmeric Trance, for Eight Months.—First Case.—Some Cause for the late Increase of Cases.—Operations in the Mesmeric Trance.

THIS disease is so common in Bengal, and attains such a magnitude, that it deserves a chapter to itself, in which it will be seen that if Mesmerism cannot prevent, it is very effectual in assisting its *removal.* These singular, and often prodigious tumours are generally called "elephantiasis of the scrotum;" but, correctly speaking, this is a misnomer, many of them not having their origin in the constitutional affection called elephantiasis, but arising from local irritation and debility of the parts, caused by syphilitic sores, or simple hydrocele; and the appearance of the tumours and aspect of the patients are often characteristic of their respective exciting causes.

In true constitutional elephantiasis the disease is accompanied with periodic fever, and general cachexy to such a degree as to make it unsafe to remove the local excrescence. The disease, in this shape, is endemic in Bengal almost exclusively, it being rarely seen in upper India, and appears to have its origin in a hot, moist, malarious, relaxing climate, in which the poor are ill-fed and ill-clothed. In Egypt it is also principally confined to the delta of the Nile, which considerably resembles Bengal in climate and the condition of its people. Endemic sources of disease abound here to a dreadful extent, but chiefly originate in the ignorance, indifference, and poverty of the people; and an enlightened and benevolent government should interfere to prevent its subjects perishing in their ignorance, by enforcing stringent police regulations for the improvement of the public health, especially by attention to drainage and filling up all unnecessary pools of water. Ragged old tanks, and offensive pools and holes of water, form a chain along the roadside, in and near all towns and villages, and spread like a network over the country; their insulation rendering them only the more pestiferous, by making each an independent hotbed of malarious exhalations. The thing is so general, that every cottage may be said to be built over a green putrefying pool, out of which the mud to build a house had been taken, and which is reckoned a *domestic convenience.* Into this all the animal and vegetable *debris* of the houses is thrown: the pigs wallow in it, the people wash their fish and rice, and bathe in it; and it is then used for cooking and drinking, as it is conveniently near, and saves the trouble of going to the nearest large tank, or the river. This accumulation of animal and vegetable matter, festering under a tropical sun, renders every hole a pest pit, and the whole population eat, drink, and breathe perpetual infection. The effects are as dreadful as might be anticipated in a debilitating climate, and among an ill-fed people, and are deeply written in the personal appearance of the natives of the country.

Ague, remittent fever, spleen, rheumatism, diarrhœa, dysentery, and cholera are inherited by the poor people along with their homes; and the general constitutional debility is evidenced by the incredible frequency of elephantiasis, diseases of the skin, and parasitic growths on the body. Ague and spleen were endemic diseases in Scotland, fifty years ago, when every cottage had its "midden" before the door; and if northern nations suffer so much from miasmatic influences, we can readily imagine their terrible energy in Bengal, where every aid and appliance is afforded them.

I shall give an illustration of the extreme gravity of these causes of disease, from a case which lately occurred in my private practice, and which I am disposed to regard as an acute form of the disease which, in its chronic shape, gives rise to constitutional elephantiasis. On the 16th May, 1845, I was requested to visit one of the richest Hindoo families here; and on going, found eight persons, men, women, and children, labouring under different degrees of the same disease, and of which two men of the same party had died, shortly before. In the worst cases the feet were swollen, and hard as in elephantiasis, and a brick-red inflammation extended half way up the leg, and was still advancing. The others were worn out with fever, and their bodies were generally or partially dropsical. The party consisted of one family and its attendants: no other persons living in the same house were affected. This led me to suspect some local cause of contamination, and I requested to be allowed to view the suite of apartments occupied by this part of the family. The house is a large two-storied pile, in which, as usual, all the family connections live. I could see nothing objectionable about the rooms inhabited by my patients; but, on looking out of the back windows, I saw that the house rose right over a large, ragged, neglected tank, covered with green filth, and smelling vilely, and that this was the only part of the house so situated. I then examined below, and perceived that the water was led upon a brick platform to a passage in the lower story, to save the people from going out; numerous narrow lanes, the sides as high as the house, led from the tank to the different parts of the house, and all opened into the court around which this family exclusively lived in small ill-ventilated rooms. In short, it was a most ingenious labyrinth, contrived for receiving and retaining all the mephitic vapours from the tank, into which were thrown all the "exuviæ" of this large family, or rather clan. This year, it so happened, was peculiarly adapted to the development of malaria; all the tanks in the district being dried up to the dregs; so that, for months, this large putrid area had been exhaling death among this unfortunate family. The disease, I therefore concluded, was only an aggravated form of the malarious fever that usually ends in elephantiasis and dropsy; the stage of elephantiasis being only more acute than usual, from constitutional peculiarity, or the severity of the disease. Being questioned as to their probability of recovery, I said, that there was little hope, except for one of them, and at this moment (1st Dec.,) one only is alive, but not recovered.

The true "elephantiasis" scrotal tumours are excessively dense in the rind, the cells of the cellular membrane being filled with dense fibrinous deposit, that makes it look and cut like half-tanned hide; the skin is black, and the mass is usually studded with tubercles.

The disease sometimes only attacks the skin of the penis; and this organ, in one instance, was as long and thick as a man's arm, and ended in a wart bigger than a fist. An incision was made down upon the penis from the symphysis pubis; and having freed it, the diseased tube was struck off where it joined the scrotum. I believe that the body of the penis will always be found unchanged and *in situ*, in this disease; the testes frequently unaltered, but very variously situated, and with common expedition, the bleeding allows time enough to save all the organs, if it is thought expedient to do so, in tumours of moderate dimensions. Even when the testes are enlarged, and castration is performed, the spermatic vessels have not their calibre or activity increased (in proof of this, I did not secure them at all in one case) ; and in general the arterial bleeding is moderate, as might be expected in a disease of a low organisation.

The mode of operating I adopt is as follows:—The penis being always *in situ*, as has been said, it is immediately found by running a bistoury from the opening in the prepuce, wherever it may be, up to the symphysis pubis, and a long *bistouri cache* is a very convenient instrument for this purpose; it is pushed up till it reaches the pubes, and the penis is exposed at once by one outward cut. The penis is then easily freed, and a semi-lunar incision carried from its root across each of the spermatic cords; these are easily found; and if the testes prove to be worth preserving, they are reflected back, the incision is extended down to the perineum on both sides, and the mass rapidly removed; if the testes are diseased, the whole is removed together. This plan is simple and expeditious: one continued wound suffices for finding the testes, and removing the tumour; and the wound has the advantage of being a gaping one, discharging the blood and water freely, and permitting one to see clearly. By this mode I always secure flaps, which often adhere in four days by the first intention; and even if they partially slough, enough is left to support and defend the testes, as they adhere to some part of the covering. The testes often adhere to the fundus of the tumour, which vexatious complication is generally caused by the natives making deep escars with the actual cautery, in the hope of discussing the swelling by suppuration; but the irritation only accelerates the disease. In these cases the spermatic cords are greatly elongated, perhaps a foot long; and they, as well as the testes, must run great risk of sloughing without any covering and natural support. In my experience, even when the flaps partially fail (I have never seen them do so entirely,) they are a great comfort to the patient by the adhesions which the cords and testes form in two or three days.

During the six years previous to April, 1845, I had operated on eleven cases; and in the last eight months, since I began to operate in the mesmeric trance, I have removed seventeen tumours, making in all twenty-eight, varying from a few pounds to eighty pounds; and there has not been a fatal case among them.

The results are—

All the parts saved in - - - - -	13
One testis sacrificed - - - - - -	6
Both - - - - - - - -	8
All removed - - - - - - -	1
	28

Of the seventeen operations in the mesmeric trance three only were imperfect, the persons awaking before the operation was finished; this imperfect sensibility was a great comfort to the patient, and gave great facilities to the operator. Here is my first case, and an example of this :—

April 23d.—Bachoo. Saw him for the first time to-day, at 11 o'clock A. M.: he has got hypertrophy of the scrotum; the tumour is twice the size of a man's head. I put him to sleep, and made his arms cataleptic in three quarters of an hour.

Pricking and inhaling ammonia disturbed, but did not awake him; I therefore proceeded to operate, but he awoke after I had slit up the prepuce. Upon this I desisted, and will try to educate him into insensibility. To be mesmerised daily.

April 27th.—He has been easily mesmerised daily, since the 23d; is not insensible to pricking, but it does not awake him, and I could afford no more time to him. I pulled him by the legs to the end of the table; allowed the tumour to hang down unsupported, and bent his knees, putting his feet on the edge of the table; and in this painful attitude he remained for half an hour, without moving. His legs and arms were then properly disposed of, in case he should awake, and the tumour quickly removed; the first incisions did not awake him, but before I was done he was completely roused.

Since then I have had *every month* more operations of this kind than take place in the native hospital in Calcutta in a year, and more than I had for the six years previous. There must be some reason for this, and I only see two ways of accounting for it: my patients, on returning home, either say to their friends similarly afflicted, "Wah! brother, what a soft man the doctor Sahib is! He cut me to pieces for twenty minutes, and I made him believe that I did not feel it. Isn't it a capital joke? Do go and play him the same trick; you have only to laugh in your elbow, and you will not feel the pain." Or they say to their brother sufferers,—"Look at me; I have got rid of my burthen, (of 20, 30,

40, 50, 60, or 80 lbs., as it may be,) am restored to the use of my body, and can again work for my bread: this, I assure you, the doctor Sahib did when I was asleep, and I knew nothing about it;—you will be equally lucky, I dare say; and I advise you to go and try; you need not be cut if you feel it." Which of these hypotheses best explains the fact my readers will decide for themselves. It ought to be added, that most of these persons were not paupers, but people in comfortable circumstances, whom no inducement short of *painless* operations could tempt to enter a charity, or any other hospital; and all who know the natives are aware of this.

I have said that only three out of the seventeen awoke before the operation was finished; I will not inflict the whole fourteen completely successful cases on the reader, but only present some of the last.

Sept. 2d.—I was stopped on the road to-day, and requested to go into a temple to see a sick Fuqueer; on entering I found a healthy-looking man of sixty, but he was nearly blind from cataracts, and had a scrotal tumour of about thirty pounds' weight, which he begged me to remove. I examined it, but gave no opinion, and said I would consider of it; I then went on to Chinsurah, to see Dr. Ross, (in charge of the troops there,) to whom I said, that if he chose to return with me, I would try to show him a mesmeric operation. He consented, and in passing the Fuqueer's house we carried him with us to the hospital. The cook of the hospital, one of my best mesmerisers, was set upon him, and in half an hour made him insensible. Considering the man's age and the size of the tumour, we did not think it worth while to attempt to save the testes, and the operation was therefore speedily done. The man never moved, and did not awake till after the last artery was tied. Seeing him about to awake, he was covered up, and asked if he had been any way disturbed; he said, "No." He was then desired to sit up, and show me the tumour, as I wished to examine it; he did so, and actually put his hands under it, to raise the mass as usual; his look of amazement, on missing it, was something not to be easily forgotten. Dr. Ross published an account of this and other operations in which he assisted me.

Oct 22d.—Muffer Dass, a peasant, aged 40. He was made insensible on the third day of mesmerising; and in the presence of Mr. Reid, the collector, Mr. Wauchope, the magistrate, and

Mr. Bennett, superintendent of Excise, I removed a tumour weighing eight pounds, without the man being disturbed; although the operation was tedious, from the testes having contracted adhesions. I succeeded in saving all the organs; he awoke soon after it was all over, said he felt no pain, and was quite ready to be operated on *now*.

Oct. 25th.—Gooroochuan Shah, a shop-keeper, aged 40. He has got a "monster tumour," which prevents him from moving; its great weight, and his having used it for a writing-desk for many years, has pressed it into its present shape. His pulse is weak, and his feet œdematous, which will make it very hazardous to attempt its removal; but with such an appendage life is literally a burthen. He became insensible on the fourth day of mesmerising, and was drawn with the mattress to the end of the bed (my usual mode of proceedings:) two men then held up the tumour in a sheet, pulling it forward at the same time, and, in the presence of Mr. Bennett, I removed it by a circular incision, expedition being his only safety. The rush of venous blood was great, but fortunately soon arrested; and, after tying the last vessel, the mattress was again pulled back upon the bed with him upon it, and at this moment he awoke. The loss of blood had been so great that he immediately fell into a fainting state, and it took a good while to remove him. On recovering he said that he awoke while the mattress was being pulled back, and that nothing had disturbed him. The tumour weighed eighty pounds, and is probably the largest ever removed from the human body. I think it extremely likely that if the circulation had been hurried by pain and struggling, or if the shock to the system had been increased by bodily and mental anguish, the man would have bled to death, or never have rallied from the effects of the operation. But the sudden loss of blood was all he had to contend against; and, though in so weak a condition, he has surmounted this, and gone on very well.

Dec. 1st.—Has been allowed to go home at his own request: the wound is filling up slowly, for want of integument.

Oct. 27th.—Rammahun Sunokur, a jeweller, aged 44, has got a large tumour. He became insensible on the fifth day, and I removed the tumour in the presence of Mr. Wauchope and Mr. Bennett. The bleeding was violent, and the testes adherent to cicatrices from burnings: I was therefore obliged to sacrifice them. About the middle of the operation he gave a cry, but did not awake till twenty minutes after it was over, and then said, that he wanted something to eat, as he felt empty. He said that he had slept well, and was not disturbed in any way; that he was now ready to be cut, but begged to be allowed to get his dinner first. The mass of flesh was now shown to him, which he recognised with amazement; thanked the gods, and said it would weigh twenty-four pounds, probably,—it weighed thirty pounds.

Nov. 2d.—Gobinchunder Lane, aged 32, a shop-keeper, and a very fine handsome man, is afflicted with the same disease.

At three o'clock yesterday, when passing the hospital, I was told that another man had come with a tumour, since my morning visit, and had been entranced. I went to see him, and found him still in a fit state to be operated on, although he had been asleep for four hours—to be mesmerised again tomorrow at ten o'clock.

Nov. 3d. The operation was performed to-day, at twelve o'clock, in the presence of the Rev. Mr. Bradbury, and Mr. Bennett. As the bleeding was moderate, and the man perfectly passive, I tried to save all the parts, although the testes adhered to the sides of the tumour, which were very thick. It was twenty minutes before all was over: not a sign of life appeared, and the organs were all saved.

Before commencing, I put his arm erect in the air as an *"oudanometer:"* it never even trembled, was quite stiff at the end of the operation, and had to be taken down. He awoke just as the mattress was readjusted, and said, "It is done!" Being asked how he knew, he said, by seeing me bloody, and the people all standing round, but that he had felt nothing, and had little pain now. The excrescence weighed twenty-five pounds.

Nov. 16th.—Ameer Mullick, a coolie, aged 50, has a large tumour of twenty years' growth. He was mesmerised for the second time to-day, and, in the presence of Mr. S. Palmer, and Dr. Scott, I dissected out, and saved all the organs. The operation was tedious, on account of old adhesions; but he did not awake till some time after it was finished, and then said, that nothing had disturbed him. The mass weighed thirty pounds.

Nov. 18th.—Bungsee, a peasant, aged 55, has a tumour which weighed twenty-eight pounds, when cut off, and has existed for nine years. He was entranced on the second day, and I removed it in the presence of Mr. Russell, Judge of Hooghly, Major Smith, H. M.'s 9th Regiment, Dr. Scott, and Captain Smythe, of the Engineers. I found all the organs, and showed that the testes were atrophied and useless; they were therefore sacrificed, and the man never moved, or showed a sign of life, till ten minutes after the operation, and he then said, that he was quite ready to be operated upon.

In concluding this practical part of the subject, I beg to state, that I have seen no bad consequences whatever ensue from persons being operated on in the Mesmeric trance. Cases have occurred in which no pain was felt, even subsequent to the operation, and the wounds healed by the first intention; and in the rest I have seen no indication of any injurious consequences to the constitution. On the contrary, it appears to me to have been saved, and that less constitutional disturbance has followed than under ordinary circumstances.

In my early operations, I availed myself of the first fit of insensibility, not knowing whether I could command it back at pleasure; and when the coma is deep enough on the first occasion, it is probably best for the patient that it should be taken advantage of, as the fewer liberties we take with Nature the better, the rule being never to do more than enough. But if the trance is not profound the first time, the surgeon may safely calculate on its being so the next, and, when operating in public, it is prudent to take the precaution of a preliminary trance or two. I have already said, that flexibility of the limbs, till moved, and their remaining rigid in any position we leave them in, is characteristic of the trance: but there are exceptions, and these are equally diagnostic and to be depended upon. It sometimes happens that the limbs become rigid as they lie, and, on bending them, they are not passive and plastic, as in the first kind of catalepsy, but the muscles always tend towards a spasmodic extension of the limbs: at other times, there is a complete relaxation of the whole muscular system, and the arms and legs can be tossed about without resistance, like those of a person just dead. The eyes are usually closed, but the eyelids are sometimes seen a little separated, or half open and tremulous; and the eye is even wide open, fixed, and the pupil dilated. On one occasion, having ordered a man to be entranced, I returned in two hours, and was told by my assistant that he was not affected: I went to see, and found him with half open eyes, quivering eye-lids, and trembling hands. I immediately said the man was ready, and, without testing his condition farther, performed on him a tedious, but painless, operation.

I also wish to remark, that I have seen no indication of congestion of blood on the brain; the circulation, while my patients were in the trance, being natural, like that of a sleeping person. Those I operate upon appear to escape the stimulating stage of the mesmeric influence altogether, and to pass at once from life to temporary death; and this I am disposed to attribute to the concentrated uninterrupted manner in which the power is applied; as soon as it is felt, there is no time given to the system to rally round the first impression, and it succumbs, without a struggle, to the constraining influence. Some patients, when suddenly awoke, say that their vision is hazy, and their heads light, but I take this to arise from the imperfectly recovered sensibility of the brain and organs of sense, which are not at once roused up to the full possession of their waking powers; just as is seen in persons suddenly aroused from profound natural sleep. That the mesmeric torpor of the nerves and brain does not arise from sanguine congestion, is often strikingly and beautifully illustrated by the first actions of persons suddenly awoke from the trance. They open their eyes wide, and at the same moment their faculties are restored, but it is seen that the pupil is dilated, and insensible to light: this they also immediately become aware of; they know that their eyes are open, and that they ought to see, but do not. The thought fills them with horror, and, with a fearful cry, they bury their faces in their hands, like persons struck blind by lightning; but this soon passes off, and the retina recovers its sensibility, by a little rubbing of the eyes.

For any person to see this, or even hear of it from a credible quarter, and still talk of imposture, is to convict himself of an incurable moral blindness, which it would be folly to attempt to dissipate by experiment and reasoning:—"none are so blind as those who *won't* see."

The dreadful shock given to the mind under such circumstances, or when a somnambulist awakens and finds himself perhaps standing naked among strangers (an experiment I have often made,) is a trial of the nerves, to which it would be very imprudent, and unsafe, to subject any but such singularly impassive beings as my patients:—sometimes, however, it is too much for the nerves of a cooly even. In highly nervous and irritable constitutions the effects might be most disastrous both to mind and body; and I would not dare to take such liberties with European temperaments. This, and the dangers and inconveniences of inducing the "Mesmeric Disease," by practising on the system *more than is necessary for the cure of disease,* appear to me to be the real dangers to be avoided in the use of Mesmerism as a remedy.

I am now able to say from experience, that debility of the nervous system predisposes to the easy reception of the mesmeric influence; and I argue favourably of the patient's powers of submission, when I recognise in him the languid, listless air that characterises functional debility of the nerves.

As I never have attempted, and never will attempt, to mesmerise people in health, I cannot speak from my own experience as to their mesmeric sensibility; but we are assured by the best authorities that many persons in health can be subdued, and my experiments go to support this. My patient Mrs. —— had not a toothache even when she was mesmerised, in order to prepare her for the dentist; and many others suffered only from some local complaint, that did not apparently impair the powers of life. The fact is sufficiently established; and experimenting on the healthy ought to be discouraged, as it is only undermining healthy constitutions for no possible advantage. The artificial disease is not so transitory or light a matter as it seems to be reckoned by many Mesmerisers, who go about upsetting the nerves of every one they can lay hands on. In proof of this I may mention, that after prisoners have been working on the roads for two or three months, I have found them still as much under my command as ever.

It is proper that ladies and gentlemen who beg to be mesmerised for fun should know this; and then they will probably choose some other kind of amusement.

CHAPTER IX.

Curiosities of Mesmerism.—Unsatisfactory Nature of Public Exhibitions.—Apology for giving one.—Account of it by a Visitor.—The Modes in which the Mesmeric Fluid can be transmitted.—It acts at great Distances.—Is absorbed by Water.—Can pass through a Wall.—Final Experiments.

My original intention was to confine myself strictly to an examination of the medical pretentions of Mesmerism, and to eschew all but the practical part at present, and thus open the minds of men to a reception of new truths, by the key of self-interest. Not that I was, by any means, indifferent to the philosophic and extra-professional bearings of the subject, but because I saw that the gross and palpable bodily phenomena, even, were more than the public stomach could bear, and I did not intend to serve up all my mesmeric stores, till the public had digested my first course of facts that cannot be denied.

But accident, if it does not determine, generally shapes our actions; and (as in my accidental *recontre* with somnambulism) I have been driven, by the force of circumstances, out of the prudent mesmeric course, which I had resolved to follow.

But as the *"utile"* has not been sacrificed to the *"dulce,"* I hope to be pardoned by the stern utilitarian reader for devoting a chapter to the *"Curiosities of Mesmerism."*

Knowing the worthlessness of public exhibitions for effecting a general conversion to the truth of Mesmerism, I was very averse to subject it to this unsatisfactory ordeal, and determined not to be made a showman of. All performers in public are not unnaturally suspected to take insurances from Art, in the event of Nature failing them; success on such occasions being thought to be more indispensable than truth. Besides this natural distrust of public displays, the really careful and intelligent observer has not the necessary means of close inspection, required to convince him beyond a doubt, and the mere sight-seer is only bewildered, and declares it to be "all humbug," because all beyond his comprehension. But in our present state of ignorance it is as absurd to pretend to set limits to the *possible* in any unexplored regions of Nature, as it would be for the inhabitants of an ant-hill in the plains of Bengal to decide authoritatively against the possible existence of the Himalayahs. I had acted with considerable consistency for some months, in confining my public mesmeric experiments to purely professional subjects; but a very general curiosity was excited, and I was at length requested, from a high quarter, to gratify some of the inhabitants of Government-House with an especial mesmeric *"Seance."* This I could hardly have refused without appearing churlish; and it would have been said that I shunned the light, because my proceedings would not bare inspection. I therefore thought it best to submit to a necessary evil, and make the most of it, by converting an exclusive party into as general and promiscuous a meeting as possible. It was therefore pretty generally made known, that all the curious might be gratified *for the first and last time* on the 29th of July. Accordingly on that day I had the honour of meeting a large assemblage of Europeans and natives at my hospitals! and as a letter appeared in the newspapers the day after, giving an account of all that was done and seen, I here insert it, as it was generally allowed to give a correct account of all that happened, and mentions the points I wish to make some observations on. Six medical men were of the party, and one of them publicly acknowledged the faithfulness of the report sent to the newspapers.

PUBLIC DISPLAY OF MESMERISM AT HOOGHLY.

To the Editor of the Englishman.

"Sir,—I esteem myself fortunate in having been present at an exhibition of the powers of Mesmerism, given by Dr. Esdaile, yesterday, to satisfy public curiosity, as it is the last opportunity of the kind likely to occur, Dr. E. having for this once only, consented to mesmerise for non-professional purposes.

"The party was very numerous, two steamers having brought the curious from Barrackpore and Calcutta; and there was a large assemblage of the European and Native residents of Hooghly and Chinsurah.

"The hospital we first went to was unfortunately small, and the room too much crowded for one to see all that was done; but what escaped me will be supplied by others, I hope, as it is desirable that all the proceedings of the day should be clearly laid before the public.

"On entering the hospital, we saw two men extended on beds, with their native mesmerisers hanging over them; but I had no time to examine their process, as Dr. Esdaile proceedd to business. He said that these two men were now under the mesmeric influence, to what extent he did not know; that they required to be operated on, and that he would do so, if they were found to be insensible.

"The first man awoke on being pulled, and called upon by name; so he would not do. The other, an elderly man, the Doctor thought was in a favourable state, and he immediately did what was needful; it is needless to say what, but every one was sure that it was very painful. The first cuts did not seem to annoy the man, but he awoke, and cried out before the operation was finished, which was a couple of minutes I suppose. The mesmeriser was desired to continue his efforts, and I saw him breathe on the head, and place both hands at the same time on the pit of the stomach; Dr. E. explaining that he often succeeded in restoring the trance, although broken to this degree. And sure enough in a few minutes, the man became perfectly senseless, to all appearance, and every body was allowed to examine and experiment upon him for the whole time we remained here; and as I believe there were several medical men present, making active observations, I hope that they will favour us with the results of their investigation. We were now agreebly surprised by the apparition of two lady philosophers, and the Doctor had to give them his attention, and certainly made them an offer they will not receive every day, for he begged them to choose whether they would prefer to see a woman made senseless by mesmeric water, or through the wall. The wall was declared for, and the woman's face turned to it sitting upon her bed.

"The Doctor disappeared, and what he did, I know not, but some went to see: whatever it was, the woman soon began to nod, and then fell down on her bed, her eyelids twinkling in a strange way, and she paid no attention to what was said to her. Dr. E. now returned from his ambuscade, having been absent for about five minutes, and pointing to the quivering eyelids, said, that this was very characteristic of the mesmeric state, and that it would be seen that this woman could not open her eyes without his assistance. After blowing in her eyes to restore her senses, she was desired, and then ordered, to open her eyes, and strained violently to do so; but the eyelids looked as if gummed together, and she could not separate them. She then, on being urged still farther, pulled the lids asunder, but they instantly closed again. Dr. E. now rubbed her eyes, and blew into them, and she immediately awoke, but in a delirious state, and arose to walk, muttering and staggering about in a singular manner; and on being taken back to bed, she fell into a deep sleep, which usually lasted four or five hours, we were told.

"We were next addressed by Dr. E., who said that he would now show us that the mesmeric power was not so rare and singular a gift as was imagined, but a general law of Nature, which might be evolved by most people who took the necessary degree of trouble; and to prove this, he would desire one of his hospital assistants to mesmerise a woman across the room, a distance of thirty feet, I should think. The woman was placed with her back to the wall, and a young man placed himself before her, at the other end of the room. In a very short time she acted exactly like the first woman; her eyes began to twinkle; she swayed from side to side, and then fell down in a trance, from which no one could awake her—not even the doctors, who again examined the man who had been operated upon before leaving, and no one succeeded, I believe, in extracting a sign of sensibility.

"We were now requested to go to another hospital, where there was more space for the company. We found it to be the Jail Hospital, where there was ample accommodation for all,—the party having tailed off considerably.

"Dr. E. said that he would attempt to show, in a more striking manner, the great distance at which the mesmeric influence could be felt. A man was brought in, and made to sit on the floor with his back to the wall, and the Doctor sat down opposite him at the other end of the room, which I afterwards measured, and found to be eighty feet long.

"We all congregated at the other end to watch the effects of this 'Long Range,' and I heard some good jokes cut, about keeping out of the line of fire, and the danger of the gun bursting, &c.

"The Doctor had proved his gun, however, I suppose, as he coolly and steadily took aim at his man, keeping his hands extended, and moving them across his face, and from head to foot. I could distinguish no sensible effects for ten minutes, and I imagine he became impatient, as he took a look at his opponent through an opera glass, and then desired him to rise, to judge of the effects, I presume. The man obeyed with great difficulty, and his tormentor, taking another look through his glass, appeared to be satisfied with his work, as he cried out to us to prevent him from falling, and not unnecessarily; for the patient trembled violently, and had to be supported. The operator now bid us move his arms, and seeing them remain in any position they were left in, declared him entranced, and being asked if we might now touch him, he called out—'Oh, yes! do what you please.' He now fell into the Doctors' hands principally, and I hope they will report the results of their criticism. I saw, however, that the man was quite insensible, and his limbs cataleptic; and that no one could excite his attention. Dr. Esdaile sat all this time alone, at the other end of the room, apparently enjoying, through his glass, the mischief and perplexity he had created. After we had extracted all we could out of this mesmeric condition of the body, Dr. E. joined us, and set about restoring him to some degree of sensibility by rubbing and blowing in his eyes. He now half opened his eyes, and followed the Doctor when led, into the middle of the room; but like a drunken man, and care had to be taken, lest he should fall. Dr. E. said that he would now convert him into an imitating machine, with only sense enough left to hear and obey his orders, without the power of answering questions; reflection being quite dormant. Having cleared up his brain a little more, and attracted his attention by repeating the key note several times, the performance proceeded. He was ordered to do what the Doctor did, and certainly obeyed his orders most exactly, throwing himself, on the instant, into every attitude of the mesmerist, and the very scientific manner in which he took a landsman's 'sight' did great credit to his astronomical powers; no omnibus cad could take the longitude of an obnoxious passenger in a more artist-like manner. His mode of cocking his eye and of applying his first digit to the side of his nose, was also much admired, and proved that he was 'wide awake,' as some thought, all the time.

"His instructor next ordered him to repeat whatever he said, which the pupil obeyed by repeating *the order*.

"He now showed himself to be a patriotic and loyal British subject, by the animated and hearty manner in which he repeated, 'Ye Mariners of England,' and sang, 'God save the King.' This was followed by "Hey diddle diddle,' in capital style. And here a curious incident occurred; the spectators could not restrain their laughter, in which the singer joined in full chorus, and some said, 'He can't help laughing himself.' Upon which Dr. Esdaile stopped his performance, and pointed out that they were labouring under a mistake who supposed that *he* was laughing; the fact being that he was only imitating them, or rather Dr. E., who was laughing '*Gorge deploye*;' and this, I think, must have been evident to all. But the farce was nearly converted into a tragedy; for on being ordered to show how the natives fight with sticks, be began very skilfully; but on bending forward to make a blow, he pitched head foremost into Dr. E.'s breast, and both rolled upon the floor. This actor's powers were clearly exhausted, and he was left in an intense trance on the floor.

"It was intimated that the next scene would be 'A Mesmeric interview; or the dangerous effect of getting on the wrong side of the wall;' and two men were brought in, and placed one in each corner of the room. Two lads were then despatched to work the will of the magician, who remained with us. This time, I was resolved to see both sides of the wall, and going into the adjacent room, I saw the two youths standing with their foreheads against the wall, opposite the men, and holding their hands extended under their mouths. In five minutes, the lads were desired to desist, and on returning to the large room, I saw the men had been turned round, and were standing perfectly rigid in their corners with their arms crucified against the wall, and in this transaction Dr. E. was no more concerned than I was. The Doctors again took possession of the victims, and I had afterwards an opportunity of taking a pull, and giving a pinch, but took nothing by my motion any more than the rest.

"Our entertainer then proclaimed that the concluding piece would be the sleeping water, or the 'veritable *eau merveilleuse.*' He said that when we saw its effects, he hoped that he would be justified for not showing in public how it was made, as it was not fit for the public to know, but that he would be happy to explain the process for the purposes of medicine and philosophy. To guard against all imposition, two Clergymen, and two Doctors, were deputed to see the water charmed, and in a few minutes half-a-dozen lads entered, each carrying a gallipot in his hands, the contents of which (certainly, to all appearance, water) he administered to eight men who were brought from the hospital.

"This was a bold undertaking, for the people were scarcely permitted to lie down before they were cuffed and kicked unmercifully, many of the company making a vigorous use of their understanding in this way.

"A few minutes comparative quiet having been procured to some of the sleeping candidates, the result was, that four out of eight were found to be cataleptic, and several were converted into somnambulists.

"I have thus endeavoured to give an account of what was

done and seen by all; but in so large a field of observation, much must have escaped me, and each person will have something distinctive and characteristic to narrate. The medical men seemed to be wide awake, and availed themselves of the opportunity; and if they have not made up their minds, it is for no want of subjects. Trusting that they will give the professional details, which I cannot supply,

"I am your obedient servant,

"A MESMERIC VISITOR.

"*Calcutta, 30th July,* 1845."

It is not merely a matter of curiosity to ascertain whether the mesmeric fluid can traverse air, and denser substances, to what distance it can be transmitted, and what circumstances assist or retard its operation.—These are all questions of great interest to the Natural Philosopher, as, by ascertaining them, he will probably detect analogies and affinities between the mesmeric fluid and other better known natural powers, and perhaps prove that it is only a modification of an inorganic agent, or a combination of several, to meet the wants of animal life; and the philosopher will naturally look to the physician for his facts, in a matter with which the latter is most conversant.

If there is a transmission of some vital product from one person to another, it must pass undeteriorated through the air, for the bodies are not in contact, and the effect, in the first instance, can be produced at a distance of an inch or several feet, and the intervals can be increased to a wonderful degree in proportion to the sensibility developed by frequent trials. An intervening *inch* of air between the two bodies being proved to be no obstacle, it is in vain to dogmatise about the possible extent of the mesmeric sphere of action; if we wish to ascertain this, it must be by actual experiment. In acting upon persons, through the air, without any gesticulations, and by the agency of water, we can make an experiment without exciting the smallest suspicion, and when these are frequently successful in *first trials,* I should think that it must be considered conclusive proof of the transmissibility of the mesmeric fluid by these media. The possibility of affecting persons in this way had never been dreamt of by my assistants; and it is needless to insist on the impossibility of my patients knowing any thing about it;—in a word, no human being could divine my intentions when I made my first attempt to mesmerise at a distance: I had not determined when or how to try it, and this was decided by an accidental favourable opportunity. In the women's ward, there is a row of pillars in the centre of the room, and it happened one day that, while leaning against the centre pillar giving some orders, I saw that the beds of the women Nobee and Alunga were on either side of me, in front, at the distance of four or five yards. The women were both sitting up in bed with their faces towards, but not looking at; me; and I seized the lucky moment to open my masked battery upon them. I first turned my looks on Alunga, and simply made her the object of my exclusive attention; her eyelids soon began to quiver, and in a few minutes she acted precisely in the manner described by my "Mesmeric Visitor." I then turned to Nobee, and she succeeded equally soon in *her way*, which never partakes of excitement; she only becomes lethargic, and passes, at once, into mesmeric sleep; and this has been done subsequently to these and other patients, by all kinds of persons, often in my absence, and as readily as by myself. The experiments have been so numerous and unexceptionable, that I must consider the transmission of the mesmeric fluid through a large body of air to be incontestably proved. This being the case, the permeability of denser materials by it might be pretty confidently expected; and he must be a person of cold imagination, who, admitting the passage of the vital fluid through the impassive air, yet stops short at a *wall* as the "ultima Thule" of his mesmeric belief, and declares all transmural agency to be *impossible!* Mineral magnetism finds no obstacle to its progress in the grossest textures, and traverses the earth from pole to pole; electricity finds its way as easily through the walls of a house as through the ambient air; and why subtile animal fluids should not be endowed, in a modified degree, with such qualities, I do not understand: it seems they must be condemned to lose their very essence probably, to gratify *our* notions of the fitness of things! But it is in vain that we presume to prescribe a course to Nature, and hedge her round with dogmas, in order to maintain our infallibility: the "Sacred College" was rapidly revolving through space, while its learned members were constraining the earth to remain a fixture by a "Senatus consultum," as had been determined by the wisdom of the schools; and the mesmeric fluid will, "like a chartered libertine," not only permeate the air, but also probably pass through walls, let its opponents oppose its progress by what arguments they please. In coming to this conclusion, I only rely on *first trials* also, and their results have been as positive and striking as any I have recorded. I have shown that a person whose system has been deeply imbued with the mesmeric action, will sometimes become entranced by merely turning his face to the wall, and leaving him quiet for a few minutes: all the account that such a mesmeric victim can give of himself is, that he feels a coldness and numbness in the limbs, a sense of weight in the back of the head, and an unconquerable heaviness of the eyelids before he goes to sleep. But I can hardly imagine that this spontaneous mesmeric paroxysm took place in *all* the numerous first trials we have made with new subjects, who had never been placed against a wall before, and to whom this position could not therefore be a source of excitement. I acknowledge the *possibility* of some of these being cases of independent Mesmerism, as the constitution, to be affected in this manner, must be deeply tainted; and something unusual was certainly done to them. To solve this doubt effectually, I have of late been looking out for a *blind* man, and one has luckily presented himself within the last few days. I have experimented on him solely for the purpose of determining the points in question, more particularly by the wall problem; and if this supplemental evidence should be still in any part open to objection, I shall be happy to repeat the examination on other blind men, till the evidence shall be considered perfect. In the mean time, I must declare myself almost satisfied, but hope that I shall be the first to change this or any other opinion here advanced, whenever contradicted by new facts.

Dec. 14th.—Janoo, a blind prisoner; he has got cataracts in both eyes, and can only distinguish light from darkness. I placed him on a stool before me to-day, and entranced him in ten minutes; I then roused him up a little, and made him a somnambulist; he walked with great difficulty, and while doing so said he was fast asleep in his bed. He very soon became unable to support himself, and fell into the trance, in which he remained for two hours.

Dec. 15th.—When sitting in the middle of the room to-day, I went and looked steadily at him from outside the window; in less than ten minutes I knocked him on the head and toes with a long bamboo, and he was quite insensible. On trying to make him walk to-day, I found there was a total dissolution of the muscular system; when placed on his feet he immediately sunk down all in a heap, and on trying to awake him it brought on an alarming fit of convulsive sobbing; on being put to bed it ceased, but again returned on my renewing attempts to awake him; he slept for more than two hours.

Dec. 16th.—I sent the Sub-Assistant Surgeon to the Jail Hospital, desiring him to get the man placed with his face towards the wall, but not touching it; to take care not to excite his attention, and to keep him engaged in conversation. I followed, and placed myself opposite him on the other side of the wall, leaning my forehead against it, and extending my hands under my mouth. In ten minutes I went to see what was done, and found him conversing in a lively manner with my Assistant: returned, and gave him five minutes more; went to see again: found them still talking, but in about two minutes he ceased to answer, and burst into a fit of convulsive crying: I now pulled him by the hair, and he fell back like a person just dead: slept for three hours.

Dec. 19th.—Mr. Samuells, the collector of Burdwan, being with me to-day, I took advantage of his presence to give this man his first dose of mesmerised water. This was prepared in a different room, and sent to him by a prisoner who usually administers the medicine, and he was ordered to give it as such; in two or three minutes he was completely insensible.

Dec. 20th.—To-day I saw him sitting in front of the cook-room, eating his dinner, and thought it a good opportunity to observe, unperceived, the extent of his blindness. The cook-rooms are about a hundred yards long, and there is a low wall in front, over which one can look kneeling: he was near one end, and I entered at the other, proceeding till I came opposite him, when I carefully observed him over the wall. He had nearly finished his dinner; and all his looks and actions convinced me that he only knew the difference of night and day. After he had washed his hands and mouth he sat chirping in the sun, as it was very cold, and seemed to feel quite comfortable; he occasionally called on some one by name, and, if answered, cracked a joke with him. I now left my ambush, and seated myself opposite to him in the open air at the distance of twenty yards; in about a quarter of an hour he raised one arm, rested his elbow on his knee, and leant his head on the hand; immediately after he supported his head on both hands on his knees, and swayed a little to one side; the inclination gradually increased (he never making an effort to rectify it) till he lost his balance, and fell head foremost into the puddle of water he had made in washing himself; his attitude was not in the smallest degree changed, and he looked like a sitting statue reversed. He was carried to bed; awoke after three hours, and asked how he had got there.

Dec. 26th.—I saw him sunning himself in front of the hospital to-day, and seated myself on the ground opposite him at the distance of thirty yards; in less than five minutes he leaned to one side, and then fell as if shot: slept for two hours.

From the foregoing facts it is allowable to conclude, I hope, that Mesmerism is a natural power of the human body.

That it affects directly the nervous and muscular systems.

That in the mesmeric trance the most severe and protracted surgical operations can be performed, without the patients being sensible of pain.

That spasms and nervous pains often disappear before the mesmeric trance.

That it gives us a complete command of the muscular system, and is therefore of great service in restoring contracted limbs.

That the chronic administration of Mesmerism often acts as a useful stimulant in functional debility of the nerves.

That as sleep, in the absence of all pain, is the best condition of the system for subduing inflammation, the mesmeric trance will probably be found to be a powerful remedy in local inflammations.

That the imagination has nothing to do with the *first* physical impression made on the system by Mesmerism, as practised by me.

That it is not necessary for the eyes to be open: I always shut them as a source of distraction; and blind men are as readily mesmerised as others.

That water can be charged with the mesmeric fluid, and has a powerful effect on the system when it has been previously affected.

That the mesmeric influence can be transmitted through the air to considerable distances, and even pass through dense materials.

APPENDIX.

When speaking of Somnambulism, I ventured to express my belief that "Clairvoyance," or the transference of sense, had been witnessed in diseased states of the body, and that, as we can imitate Nature step by step, by artificially producing Somnambulism, Catalepsy, and a state of the system resembling Hysteria, in which "Clairvoyance" has been witnessed as a symptom in disease; so we might expect to see this phenomenon in the analogous derangements of the nervous system brought about by Mesmerism. It ought to be remembered that this is one of the wonders of Nature, and also, a great rarity in art, and must not be looked for, as a matter of course, in persons under the influence of Mesmerism. It has not yet fallen under my observation, and from want of books, I could not present the reader with as many well-attested proofs of its existence in Nature as was desirable.

After the foregoing work was finished, I fortunately met Professor Wienholt's "Lectures on Somnambulism," and, as I there found all the facts required to establish the existence of natural Clairvoyance, and, in the notes of the learned translator, Mr. Colquhoun, a parallel array of these "stubborn things" in proof of the truth of Mesmeric Clairvoyance, I hope the reader will be glad to have this additional aid to his judgment in coming to a decision. Professor Wienholt, in describing natural Somnambulism, says:

"The sleep-walker, when otherwise healthy, falls, at a particular period, into a common sleep, which cannot be distinguished from the natural state of repose. After a longer or shorter time he rises from his couch, and walks about the room—sometimes about the house. He frequently goes out into the open air, walks upon known or unknown paths as quickly, and with as much activity and confidence, as in his waking state, avoids all obstacles which may stand, or have been designedly placed in his route, and makes his way along rugged paths, and climbs dangerous heights, which he would never have thought of attempting when awake. He reads printed and written papers, writes as well and correctly as in his waking state, and performs many other operations requiring light and the natural use of the eyes. All these actions, however, are performed by the Somnambulist in complete darkness as well as when awake, and, generally, with his eyes firmly closed. I shall afterwards speak of the exceptions, in which these persons have their eyes open. When the period of his somnambulism has elapsed, he returns to his bed, falls back again into his natural sleep, awakes at his usual hour, and, in most instances, knows nothing of what he had done in his *sleep-walking* state. At the same time, there are very few persons who exhibit all of these phenomena, or even the greater number of them. For the most part, they only wander about without any other peculiar manifestation; and the instances in which several of the phenomena in question are exhibited are rare. This state, which is found in persons otherwise healthy, frequently occurs in diseases, especially in diseases of the nervous system. In the latter case, the affection usually commences with a paroxysm of convulsive motions, catalepsy, apparent syncope, and then passes over into a state precisely similar, so far as regards the principal symptoms, to Somnambulism; only that in this latter case, the patients not only act, but speak, which rarely happens in the former. Before these patients are completely restored to their ordinary waking state, their sleep is changed into a similar convulsive state, combined with want of consciousness.

"Of this species of Somnambulism occurring in nervous diseases, we are in possession of many curious instances, of which the Aulic Councillor Meiners, a celebrated professor at Goettingen, has inserted several very remarkable examples in his instructive collection. In respect to its chief characteristics, this species of Somnambulism, occurring in nervous diseases, completely resembles the natural crisis; it is recognized by all competent judges as of the same kind, and is comprehended under the same class of diseases; and in this view I also consider it. I begin with the case in Moritz's Magazine, which was first translated by Mr. Spalding, and afterwards inserted by Meiners in his collection. This is a case of what has been called 'louping ague,' which, unquestionably, is just one instance of that species of Somnambulism which I have referred to as occasionally accompanying nervous diseases. The patient was a female of sixteen years of age. The paroxysm attacked her in the morning, and consisted of a profound sleep. In this state, she would jump with astonishing activity upon tables and chairs, run, when permitted, and with great rapidity, out of the house,—generally to a particular place in the neighbourhood; and when she did not awake, she would return immediately, but sometimes by a different road, and in a different direction. She not unfrequently left the high road, and ran straight through the fields. She never fell nor injured herself, however rough her path might be, or however fast she might run; and her speed was sometimes so great, that her much stronger and more active brother could not keep pace with her. She frequently mounted upon the garden wall, upon the uneven top of which she continued to run; nay, she even went upon the edge of the house roof without once stumbling, much less falling. *During all these hazardous operations, her eyes were fast closed, and she appeared to be deprived of all her other senses.*"

The second volume of Moritz's Magazine contains the history of a boy of nine years of age, who frequently fell into a species of Somnolency, during which he was capable of carrying on a conversation. *His eyes were fast closed, but, notwithstanding this circumstance, he saw and named all objects that were presented to him.*

A very remarkable case was related to me by a most trustworthy observer, the late Hamburgh Physician, Dr. Schulz, from whom the Aulic Counsellor Meiners, of Goettingen, also received it, and inserted it in his well-known collection. It was that of a girl between twelve and thirteen years of age, belonging to a family of some distinction, who was afflicted with a violent nervous complaint, in which strong convulsive motions alternated with catalepsy and syncope. Besides, she frequently had paroxysms, during which she conversed with much liveliness and ingenuity. *In this state, she distinguished without difficulty all colours that were presented to her, recognised the numbers of the cards, and the stripes upon those which were variegated. She described the binding of books when shown to her. She wrote in the same manner as usual, and cut figures on paper, as she was accustomed to do for pastime in her waking state. Her eyes, at this time, were firmly closed; but in order to be assured that she made no use of them, a bandage was placed over them on the approach of the paroxysm.*

Another very remarkable case will be found in the "Breslau Medical Collections." It relates to a rope-maker, who was frequently overtaken by sleep, even in the daytime, and in the midst of his usual occupations. While in this state, he sometimes recommenced doing all that he had been engaged in during the previous part of the day; at other times he would continue the work in which he happened to be engaged at the commencement of the paroxysm, and finished his business with as great ease and success as when awake. When the fit overtook him in travelling, he proceeded on his journey with the same facility, and almost faster than when awake, without missing the road or stumbling over any thing. In this manner he repeatedly went from Nuremburg to Weimar. Upon one of these occasions he came into a narrow lane where there lay some timber. He passed over it regularly without injury; and with equal dexterity he avoided the horses and carriages that came in his way. At another time, he was overtaken by sleep just as he was about to set out for Weimar on horseback. He rode through the river Ilme, allowed his horse to drink, and drew up his legs to prevent them getting wet; then passed through several streets, crossed the market-place, which was, at that time, full of people, carts and booths, and arrived in safety at the house of an acquaintance, where he awoke. These and many similar acts, requiring the use of the eyes, he performed in darkness, as well as by daylight. *His eyes, however, were firmly closed, and he could not see when they were forced open and stimulated by light brought near them.* His other senses appeared to be equally dormant as were his eyes. He could not smell the most volatile spirit. He felt nothing when pinched, pricked, or struck. He heard nothing when called by his name, or even when a pistol was discharged close beside him.

There is another case, somewhat older, observed and circumstantially reported by a trustworthy physician, Dr. Knoll, which equally deserves our attention. The subject of his observation was a young man, a gardener, who became somnambulous, and while in that state performed many extraordinary operations. He generally fell asleep about eight o'clock in the evening, and then began to utter devotional sentences and prayers. Afterwards he went out of the house, clambered over a high wooden partition, and a still higher wall, uninjured, passed through several streets, and returned. At another time he climbed up to the roof of the house, and rode astride upon the gutter, as if upon horseback, clambered about for some time upon the roof, and, at length, descended in safety. With a view to prevent accidents, he was locked up in a room, and watched. When he became somnambulous, at the usual time, he began to perform all sorts of operations on his clothes and the furniture of the room. He climbed up to the window sill, and from thence to a stone which was much higher, and at some distance, and rode upon the latter, as if upon a horse. The height of the stone, its distance from the window, and its small breadth, were such, that a person awake would scarcely have ventured to attempt these operations. After descending from the stone, he knocked a large table about hither and thither, and finding it was likely to fall on him, he very dexterously contrived to evade it. He gathered together all the clothes he could find in the room, mixed them together, then separated them carefully, and hung them up, each article in its proper place. The old stockings and shoes he endeavoured to arrange in pairs, according to their shape and colour, as if he actually saw them. He then laid hold of a needle, which he had stuck into the wall some weeks before, and sewed his small-clothes. Besides these, he performed a variety of other operations, *all requiring light and the use of the eyes, with which, it would appear, he was enabled to dispense.*

In addition to the foregoing instances, I must here notice two remarkable cases, which were both observed with great accuracy by individuals who are elevated far above all suspicion of credulity, deceit, and imposture. The one is reported by the Professor, and Aulic Counsellor, Feder. The subject of his observations was a student, who, during a severe nervous complaint, experienced several attacks of Somnambulism. Upon these occasions he would go from his bed-room to his parlour and back, open and shut the doors, as well as his closet, and take out of the latter whatever he wanted—pieces of music, pen, ink, and paper, *and all this with his eyes shut!* From among his music he selected a march from the opera of *Medea,* laid the sheet in a proper situation before him, and having found the appropriate key, he played the whole piece with his usual skill upon the harpsichord. In the same manner he also played one of Bach's sonatas, and gave the most expressive passages with surprising effect. One of the persons present turned the notes upside down: this he immediately perceived, and when he commenced playing, he replaced the sheet in its proper position. When playing, he remarked a string out of tune, upon which he stopped, put it in order, and again proceeded. He wrote a letter to his brother, and what he wrote was not only perfectly rational, but straight and legible. While Professor Feder was on a visit to him one afternoon, he (the somnambulist) observed that it was snowing, which was actually the case. On the same occasion, *notwithstanding his eyes were still completely closed,* he remarked that the landlord of the opposite house was standing at the window, which was true, and that hats were hanging at the window of another room, which was also the fact. He opened Professor Feder's *Compendium* of logic and metaphysics, and pointed out to him several passages which he thought interesting, as also some of his own written notes of the Professor's lectures in a volume which had been recently bound. We must observe, however, the remarkable circumstance—common to him, indeed, with several other somnambulists—that there were many things he did not perceive. Thus, while writing to his brother, he did not observe that there was no more ink in the pen, and continued to write on. At one time he struck fire, and held the tinder to his ear, as if to hear the crackling, and then ascertain if it was burning. He lighted a match, came to the candle, and held it in the middle of the flame.

In conclusion, I may refer to the case observed by the Archbishop of Bourdeaux, and reported in the great French Encyclopedia. It is the case of a young ecclesiastic, in the same seminary with the Archbishop, who was in the habit of getting up during the night in a state of Somnambulism, of going to his room, taking pen, ink, and paper, and composing and writing sermons. When he had finished one page of the paper on which he was writing, he would read over what he had written and correct it. Upon one occasion, he had made use of the expression *ce divin enfant.* In reading over the passage, he changed the adjective *divin* into *adorable.* Perceiving, however, that the pronoun *ce* could not stand before the word *adorable,* he added to the former the letter *t.* In order to ascertain whether the somnambulist made really any use of his eyes, the Archbishop held a piece of pasteboard under his chin, to prevent him from seeing the paper on which he was writing; but he continued to write on without appearing to be incommoded in the slightest degree.

The paper on which he was writing was taken away; but the somnambulist immediately perceived the change. He wrote pieces of music while in this state, and in the same manner *with his eyes closed.* The words were placed under the musical notes. It happened, upon one occasion, that the words were written in too large a character, and did not stand precisely under the corresponding notes. He soon perceived the error, blotted out the part, and wrote it over again with great exactness.

I hope that these examples, to which I might add a great many others, will be sufficient to show that the somnambulist, during this extraordinary state, is enabled, apparently without the use of his eyes, to receive impressions equally well, or, at least, with the same consequences to his perceptive faculty, as when awake.

Mr. Colquhoun, the translator of Wienholt, supplies us from his extensive reading, with a number of the best authenticated cases descriptive of the same condition of things in Somnambulism, and derangement of the nervous system induced by Mesmerism; and as this is the only physical symptom of any consequence, described by European Mesmerists, which I have not yet seen in India, I hope that Mr. Colquhoun will excuse my making such free use of his facts, in order to complete this subject.

The reporters of the facts in question are, for the most part, men whose intellectual attainments, in general, are known to have been of a superior order, and whose moral character is elevated far above suspicion; men, in short, far more honourable and trustworthy than their wretched, chiefly anonymous, calumniators. They will be found to be, principally, eminent physicians, such as Hufeland, physician to the king of Prussia; Steiglitz, physician to the king of Hanover; Brandis, physician to the king of Denmark; Klein, physician to the king of Wirtemberg; Wienholt; Olbers, the astronomer; Gmelin; Heinecken; Bockman; Baehrens; Ennemmoser; Sprengel, author of a history of medicine, and other learned works; Haindorf; Nolte; Spindler; Nasse; Nees von Esenbeck; Passavant; Ziermann; Heinroth; Leupoldt, &c.—Physiologists, such as Reil; Treviranus; Autenrieth; Humboldt; Burdach; Eschenmayer; Kieser, &c.—Naturalists, such as La Place, Cuvier, Oken, &c.—Philosophers, such as Fichte, Schelling, Steffens, Baader, Hegel, &c.—Theologians, such as Schleiermacher, Mayer, &c. To these might be added a vast number of men of general science, and celebrated literary characters. The French magnetists—Puysegur, Deleuze, Bertrand, Georget, Cuvier, Despine, Rostan, Husson, Filassier, Foissac, Gauthier, Teste, &c.—constitute a perfect host.

But it has been alleged that the evidence of these enlightened individuals is liable to discredit, because, forsooth, they were engaged in investigating the phenomena of animal magnetism. Assuredly, this is a strange, and we must take the liberty of saying, a most preposterous objection. Pray, how are the facts of nature to be discovered and appreciated, unless by those who take an interest in investigating them? Are the facts of chemistry to be discredited, because they have been discovered by chemists? And is the same *ultra* sceptical test to be applied to electricity, galvanism, astronomy, and general physics? Are no facts to be relied upon as genuine, but such as may happen to be adduced by ignorant and unskilful persons, who have neither the requisite talent, nor the disposition for investigation, and who are, moreover, careless and indifferent to the results?

The Author, then, feels no hesitation in appealing to the experience of the most eminent magnetists, in confirmation of the fact which, as we have seen, has been manifested in many instances, of the natural Somnambulism; but in order to deprive the most obdurate sceptics of every pretence for denying the reality of the fact in question, we shall proceed to the brief enumeration of cases, in which the controverted phenomenon was distinctly and unequivocally manifested.

Dr. Tritschler's somnambulist—a boy of thirteen years of age—saw and recognised the numbers and pictures on cards, when introduced under the bedcover, and placed upon his stomach, in complete darkness, and covered, moreover, by the hand of the magnetiser. The same recognition took place in the case of written notes.

Madame Millet, magnetised by Van Ghert, saw her physician's hand and finger by means of the *epigastrium*. At a later period she recognised, in a similar manner, some portraits. At last she became so *clairvoyante* as to be able to read, by means of the *epigastrium*, at the distance of a foot and a half.

Miss St., under the care of Dr. Lehmann, accurately distinguished the colours of cards by means of the epigastrium. Kieser's epileptic boy read fluently by means of the pit of the stomach. Maria Rubel, in Langenberg, read sealed letters by means of the epigastrium; nay, even written characters enveloped in a covering of double linen. De Valenti's patient described the ornamental devices on his watch; she also recognised the picture of a soldier placed on her stomach. In many other patients the functions of other organs were also manifested at the *epigastrium*. Dr. Joseph Frank's patient, Louisa Baerkmann, recognised and felt the taste of sugared water at the epigastric region, and *heard* at the same place. A servant girl, magnetised by De Valenti, also heard at the *epigastrium*. Dr. Klein's patient said, "This is very comical—I hear by means of my stomach;" and she laughed aloud at the singularity of the phenomenon. Her ears having been stopt, she said, "That is of no use; I hear with this," pointing to her stomach.

In the case of other somnambulists, the common sense seemed to be transferred to the points of the fingers, as in the case of Miss M'Evoy, of Liverpool, Professor Kieser's patient, Anthony Arst, read with his forefinger, and distinguished cards in the same manner. Nay, when he held his elbow out of the window, he saw every thing in the street to the distance of 150 paces. Van Ghert's somnambulist saw by the means of the fingers; as also Madame Millet and Maria Rubel, formerly noticed, and Dr. Durr's patient. An idio-somnambulic boy at Halmstadt, in Holland, read fluently by means of his breast and fingers. Dr. Meyer's patient, at Dulken in Rhenish Prussia, heard with the points of his fingers. One of Dr. Kerner's somnambulists heard sometimes with her fingers, sometimes with every part of her body. Articles of food she tasted with her fingers, as with her mouth. The second somnambulist, mentioned in the work referred to, saw only when she placed her finger on the pit of the stomach, or on the crown of the head. She sometimes heard, smelt, and saw with the point of the middle finger.

Other cases are recorded in which the patients saw and heard with the nose, the chin, the elbows, the knees, the toes, and all the prominent parts of the body. Augusta Miller of Carlsruhe saw with her forehead, her eyelids, and her eye-brows. Dr. Werner mentions, as a singular peculiarity, that his somnambulist possessed the power of changing the *focus* of vision at pleasure. In some cases, it would appear, the whole body becomes as it were *clairvoyant*. This was the case with Dr. Heinecken's patient at Bremen, who saw without the assistance of the eyes, or of any other special organ; and she expressly declared that such somnambulists were much more *clairvoyant* than those whose perceptive faculties were localised. Hence the somnambulists are frequently unable to give any adequate description of these *metastases* of the perceptive faculties and the species of perception, in these cases, might, perhaps, be more properly denominated feeling, than actual *sight, hearing,* &c. It is worthy of remark, too, that the perceptions of these somnambulists, in general, are much more vivid, acute, and delicate, than in the waking state.

The foregoing observations, it is presumed, must be sufficient to convince every candid and unprejudiced mind of the existence in certain states of the organism, of the phenomenon of sensible perception, without the use of the appropriate organs.

Here, then we have a body of evidence in support of the existence of natural and artificial "clairvoyance," given by the same description of persons; physicians of eminence and unimpeached honour, a body of men who, perhaps more than the members of any other profession, are dependent on their characters as the means of winning daily bread. It appears to me, that there is no ground for preferring the evidence of one set of witnesses to the other, and that both are by their character and knowledge eminently entitled to our belief, unless we reject all human testimony, declare clairvoyance to be a subject on which it is useless to accumulate facts and evidence, and "taboo" its consideration by the human mind.

THE END.